AEPSi™ Administrator Guide

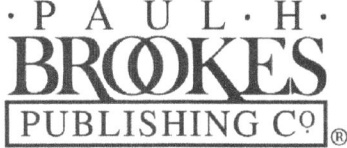

Baltimore • London • Sydney

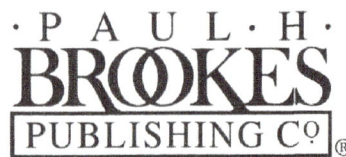

Paul H. Brookes Publishing Co.
Post Office Box 10624
Baltimore, MD 21285-0624

www.brookespublishing.com

Copyright © 2013 by Paul H. Brookes Publishing Co., Inc.
All rights reserved.

"Paul H. Brookes Publishing Co." is a registered trademark of
Paul H. Brookes Publishing Co., Inc.

"AEPS®" is a registered trademark and AEPSi™, AEPS ™, and AEPSi ™ are trademarks of Paul H. Brookes Publishing Co., Inc.

Manufactured in the United States of America by
Bradford & Bigelow, Newburyport, Massachusetts.

No real personal information is represented in any text or illustration in this guide. Any relation to true personal information is coincidental, and no inferences are intended.

For technical support for AEPSi, please call 1-866-386-2666 or e-mail techsupport@brookespublishing.com.

To contact the AEPSi Implementation Team, please e-mail implementation@brookespublishing.com.

For information regarding training, please call 1-866-386-2666 ext. 2 or e-mail seminars@brookespublishing.com.

To renew your AEPSi subscription or for customer service inquiries, please call 1-800-638-3775.

Version 1.1

ISBN-13: 978-1-59857-391-6
ISBN-10: 1-59857-391-8

2017
10   9   8   7   6   5   4   3

Contents

Introduction 1
    Welcome to AEPSi 1
    About the *AEPSi™ Administrator Guide* 1

Section 1: Managing Your AEPSi Account 2–6
    Left Menu Navigation 2
    Program Administration Home Page 3
    Program Profile 4–6
       • Classrooms 4
       • Delete Child Profiles Setting 4–5
       • Subscription Details 5
       • Account Status 5
       • Subscription Alert Messages 6

Section 2: Managing Users 7–18
    Roles and Rights Management 7–8
    Manage Administrators 8–11
       • Creating a New Administrator 8–9
       • Editing an Administrator Profile 10
       • Deactivating/Reactivating/Deleting an Administrator 10–11
    Manage Reviewers 11–13
       • Creating a New Reviewer 11–12
       • Editing a Reviewer Profile 12
       • Deactivating/Reactivating/Deleting a Reviewer 12–13
    Manage Providers 13–17
       • Creating a New Provider 14
       • Editing a Provider Profile 15
       • Deactivating/Reactivating/Deleting a Provider 15
       • Assigning Children to Providers 16–17
       • Removing Children Assigned to a Provider 17
    Assigning User Dual Roles 18

Section 3: Managing Your Children 19–33
    Creating a Child Record 19–20
    Custom Fields 20–28
       • Creating Custom Fields 21–28
          ▪ Custom Field Options 22–23
          ▪ Creating a Text Custom Field 23
          ▪ Creating a Number Custom Field 24
          ▪ Creating a Date Custom Field 25
          ▪ Creating a Yes/No Custom Field 26
          ▪ Creating a Dropdown Menu Custom Field 27–28
       • Edit/Delete a Custom Field 28
    Updating a Child's Team 29–31
       • Assigning Providers to Children 29
       • Removing Providers from a Child's Team 30
       • Creating a Caregiver Profile 30
       • Edit/Delete Caregiver Profile 31

Archiving/Deleting a Child Record	32–33
• Archiving a Child Record	32
• Reactivating an Archived Child Record	32
• Deleting a Child Record	33

Section 4: My Reports — 34–49

Child Reports	34–38
• Score Summary	35
• Graphed Scores	36
• Child Progress Record	37
• Provider Notes	37
• IFSP/IEP Summary	38
• Eligibility Cutoff Scores Report	38
• Present Level of Functioning	38
Aggregate Reports	39–49
• Class Reports Page	39
• Program Reports Page	39–40
• Group Snapshot Reports	40–42
▪ Status of All Children Report	40
▪ Progress of All Children Report	41
▪ Child Profile List Report	42
• OSEP Categories Reports	43–48
▪ About OSEP Reporting	43
▪ Children on the Alternative Path	44
▪ Entry Data Only (Aggregate Percentages) Report	44–45
▪ Entry Data Only (Categories for Each Child) Report	45
▪ Progress Data (Aggregate Percentages) Report	46
▪ Progress Data (Categories for Each Child) Report	46
▪ OSEP Report Exclusion Categories	47–48
• ECO Child Outcomes Summary Form Ratings	48–49
▪ Entry Data Only (Ratings for Each Child) Report	48
▪ Progress Data (Ratings for Each Child) Report	49

Section 5: Broadcast Messages — 50–51

Creating a Message	50
Viewing/Editing/Deleting a Message	51
Adding a Hyperlink to a Message	51

Section 6: Exporting Data — 52

Export Child Data	52
Export Program Data	52

Section 7: Support and Training — 53–55

Password Management	53
• Forgotten Passwords	53
• Forgotten Username	53
• Change Password	53
• Password Protection	53
Technical Support	54
My Toolkit	54
Online Help and Support	54
Training	55
• Customized On-Site Training	55

Introduction

Welcome to AEPSi

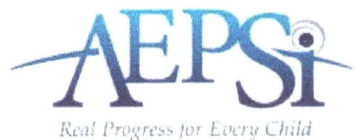

AEPSinteractive™ (AEPSi™) is a web-based management system for the *Assessment, Evaluation, and Programming System for Infants and Children (AEPS®), Second Edition,* that makes it easier for AEPS users to make the most of AEPS, meet reporting mandates, determine eligibility, and manage and track child data. AEPSi has all the integrity of AEPS plus the time- and paperwork-saving convenience of automated scoring and powerful functionality that transforms AEPS findings into Child Progress Reports and OSEP Child Outcomes Reports. Depending on individual state requirements, AEPSi can also help determine whether a child is eligible for services based on the results of the AEPS Test. AEPS is truly a complete solution for programs that also need to meet accountability and eligibility challenges—without sacrificing quality programming and good outcomes for children.

AEPSi makes it easier for you and your program to help children make real progress.

About the *AEPSi™ Administrator Guide*

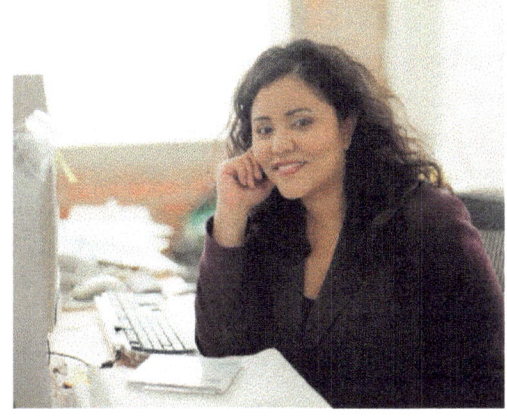

The *AEPSi™ Administrator Guide* will take you through all the steps necessary to successfully manage your AEPSi account. You will learn how to navigate the Administrator interface and manage the users and children in your program. AEPSi has simple-to-use rights management features that will enable you to specify access rights to child records as well as reporting functions for each user in the program.

In addition to creating individual Child, Class, and Program Reports, the *AEPSi™ Administrator Guide* will show you how to create automated, one-click OSEP reports based on an empirically validated crosswalk between AEPS and OSEP Indicators #3 (Part C) and #7 (Part B, Section 619).

This guide also provides information on additional training, professional development, online support and help, the discussion board, and several other resources that will prove very useful to you as an Administrator.

Thank you for choosing AEPSi as your online assessment and intervention tool.

Managing Your AEPSi Account

Section 1

When you log in to your AEPSi account, you will be taken to your **My AEPSi** page. From the **My AEPSi** page, you are able to see news and updates posted by Brookes Publishing Co. (the developer of AEPSi) under the **What's New** section; access any messages posted by your program and/or Enterprise program under **Messages**; and have quick links to any Child, Class, or Program Reports under **My Reports**.

The tabs along the top of the page allow you to navigate to different sections of the site. The tab on the far left is the **Admin** tab—this will take you to a section of the site specific to AEPSi Administrators, where you will be able to access all of the features that allow you to manage your AEPSi account.

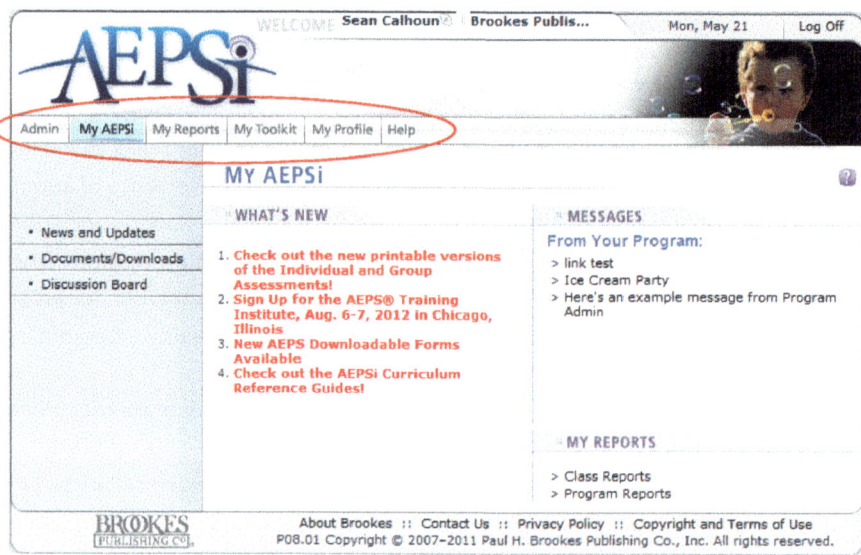

When you click the **Admin** tab, you will be taken to your **Program Administration** home page. On this page, you have quick access to the information you need to manage your AEPSi account, including help documentation and information about your program and subscription details, as well as the ability to search for users and children in your account.

Left Menu Navigation

The left menu contains links to all of the different areas within the **Admin** section. You will be able to access this same menu from any area of the **Admin** section.

The area you are currently in will be highlighted in bold.

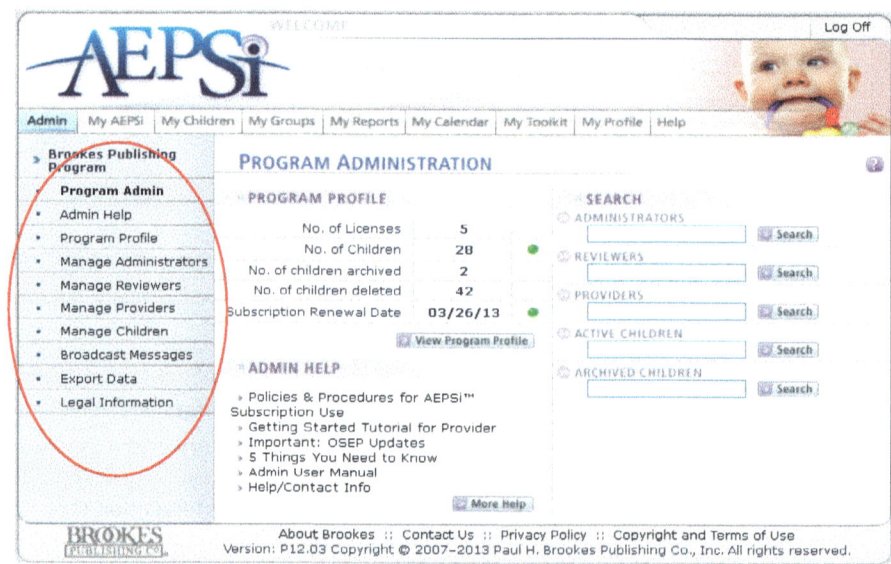

Program Administration Home Page

The content on your **Program Administration** home page offers you a quick and easy way to access the information you need to manage your AEPSi account. At the top left you will see the **Program Profile**, which displays the number of licenses purchased for your subscription, the current number of active child records in your AEPSi account, the current number of archived child records in your AEPSi account, the number of child records that have been deleted in your AEPSi account for the current subscription year, and the subscription renewal date. Next to the number of child records and subscription renewal date, there may be a blinking alert icon. The AEPSi system will provide the following alert messages:

- Number of Children:
  When the number of current active child records exceeds the number of child licenses by more than 20%, you will see a blinking alert light. Your program may receive an invoice to pay for those additional child records at that time, or the additional child records may be reconciled when it is time to renew your subscription.

- Subscription Renewal Date:
  You will see a blinking alert light 90, 60, and 30 days before it is time to renew your subscription.

> *Note: Exceeding your number of child licenses purchased will **not** result in losing access or functionality to the site.*

You can view your full program profile by clicking the *View Program Profile* button.

To the right of the Program Profile Summary is the *Search* function. To search for an Administrator, Reviewer, Provider, or child in your program, type the first name or last name in the corresponding search field and click the *Search* button. This will pull up a link to that person's profile. You can also search for a Child Profile by entering the Child ID in the search field.

The last section is **Admin Help**. Here you will find the tutorial for getting started with AEPSi, the Admin User's Manual, and a quick link for help/contact information. Clicking the *More Help* button, or clicking the *Admin Help* link on the left menu navigation, will take you to more help options.

Program Profile

To view the **Program Profile**, you can either click the *View Program Profile* button on your **Program Administration** home page, or click *Program Profile* on the left menu navigation in the **Admin** section. The **Program Profile** will display the name of the program, program type, address, city, state, and zip. In addition, there are optional fields for the phone number, fax number, and website address.

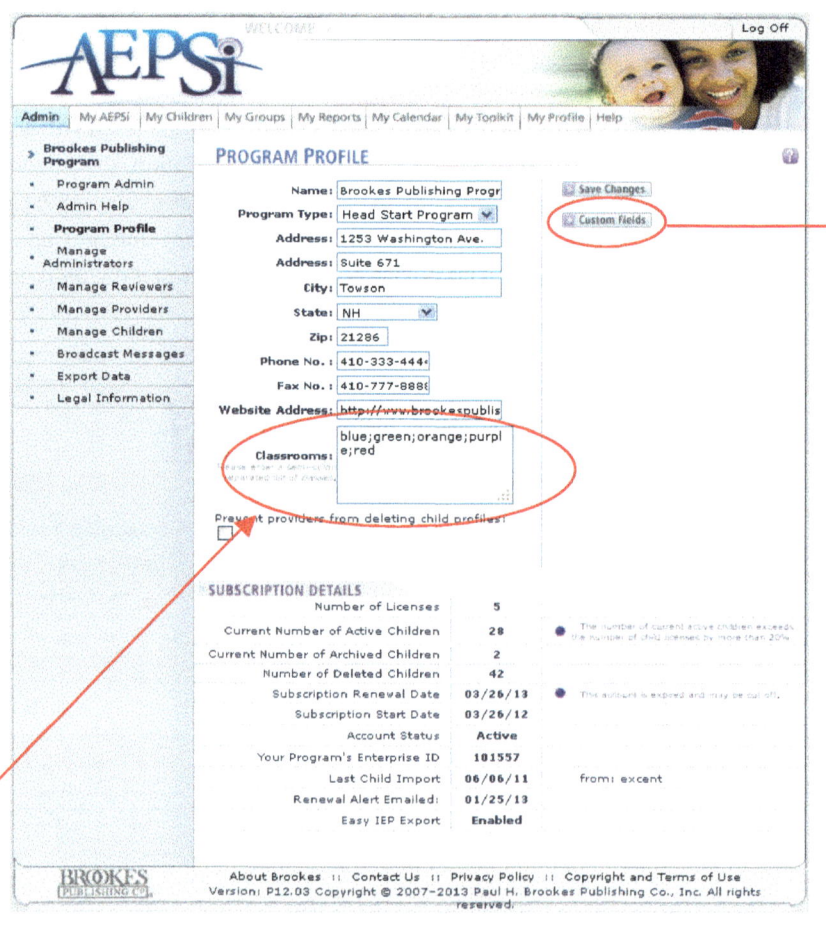

Most of this information will be completed for you when you start your subscription, but you may make any additions or changes by entering information in these text fields and clicking the *Save Changes* button.

Classrooms

Another field in the **Program Profile** is classrooms. You have the option to create classrooms by entering classroom names in the text area, separated by semi-colons. The classrooms you create will appear in a dropdown menu in the Child Profile and certain report request forms.

When an Administrator or user creates a child record, he or she can assign the child to a classroom from the dropdown menu.

The classroom dropdown menu will also appear when creating reports, which allows your users to create group reports for a particular class. There is no limit to how many classrooms can be created.

> Note: You will learn more about the Classrooms field in **Section 3: Managing Your Children** and **Section 4: My Reports**.

The **Program Profile** page is also where you can create custom fields to add to a child's profile. You will learn how the custom fields work in **Section 3: Managing Your Children**.

Delete Child Profiles Setting

As an Administrator, you have the ability to prevent Providers from deleting child profiles. This is a safeguard to make sure child data is not deleted by accident. If you do not want Providers to have the ability to delete child profiles, click the checkbox next to "Prevent providers from deleting child profiles." If the checkbox is unchecked, Providers will be able to delete child profiles.

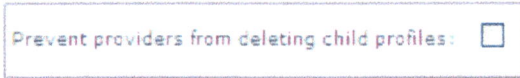

If your program is part of an Enterprise account, the Enterprise Administrator also has the ability to prevent providers from deleting child profiles. If the Enterprise Administrator has selected this option, you will see the following message on your **Program Profile** page:

"The option to prevent Providers from deleting child records has been selected by your Enterprise Administrator."

Subscription Details

The **Program Profile** page also contains details about your AEPSi subscription. That information includes:

- Number of Licenses: The number of child records purchased for the current subscription year.
- Current Number of Active Children: The current number of active child records in your AEPSi account (those not archived or deleted). This number will be updated whenever a new child record is created, as well as when a child record is archived or deleted.
- Current Number of Archived Children: The current number of archived child records in your AEPSi account. This number will also be updated whenever a child record is archived or when an archived child record is deleted or reactivated.
- Number of Deleted Children: The number of child records that have been deleted during the current subscription year. Only children for whom an assessment has been created will be included.
- Subscription Renewal Date: The date when it is time to renew your subscription. Well in advance of this date, you or the responsible party will want to contact Customer Service to renew your subscription.
- Subscription Start Date: The start date of your AEPSi current subscription period.
- Account Status: Your account status will display as one of the following: active, expired, inactive, or locked.
- Your Program's Enterprise ID: If your program is part of a larger Enterprise group, your Enterprise ID Number will be displayed here.
- Last Child Import: The date and file type of the last child imported into your program from another source.
- Renewal Alert E-mailed: The date the last e-mail was sent to your program's administrator(s) to notify you that it is time to renew your subscription.
- Easy IEP Export: If your program has opted to have access to the Easy IEP Export feature—found under the Program Reports page of your **My Reports** section—this field will read "enabled."

Account Status

Below is a brief description of the possible values for account status:

- Active: Your account is active and functional.
- Expired: Your subscription has expired, and you have not renewed your subscription. All users still have access to your AEPSi account, but you must renew your subscription immediately.
- Inactive: You have cancelled your AEPSi account. Users will no longer be able to access your account.
- Locked: Your AEPSi account has been locked, and users are unable to access the account. When an account is locked, it means that payment for subscription renewal is past due. Once the subscription has been renewed, the account will be made active again, and users will be able to access the account.

*Note: Exceeding your number of child licenses purchased will **not** result in losing access or functionality to the site.*

Subscription Alert Messages

The AEPSi system will provide the following alert messages on the **Program Profile** page:

- Current Number of Active Children: When the number of current active children exceeds the number of child licenses by more than 20%, you will receive an alert message. Your program may receive an invoice to pay for those additional child records at that time, or the additional child records may be reconciled when it is time to renew your subscription.

- Subscription Renewal Date: You will receive an alert message 90, 60, and 30 days before it is time to renew your subscription. You also will be alerted when your account has expired and you are in danger of losing access to the site.

Managing Users

Section 2

In this section, you will become familiar with the roles (Administrator, Reviewer, and Provider) and rights available for users of the AEPSi system. You also will learn how to create, edit, deactivate/reactivate, and delete users, as well as to assign Providers to children.

Roles and Rights Management

Assigning roles and permissions in AEPSi is simple. AEPSi comes with three predefined roles (Administrator, Provider, and Reviewer). You can assign one or more roles to each user in your program.

Administrator
As your program's designated AEPSi Administrator, you manage all the records and the rights of other AEPSi users in your program. Users who are Administrators can create, edit, and deactivate user records; create, archive, and delete child records; assign Providers to children and vice versa; and create reports.

Provider
The Provider role is designed for users who work directly with children, such as teachers and therapists. Users who are Providers have the ability to create and edit child records, enter assessment data, view reports on the individual children to whom they are assigned, and create Class Reports.

Within the Provider role there is a designated "Lead Provider" for each child's team. The Lead Provider is able to assign Providers to the child's team, remove Providers from the child's team, add/edit Caregiver information, and designate another Lead Provider for a child's team. Besides Administrators, only Lead Providers are able to make changes to a child's team.

Reviewer
The Reviewer role is designed for users such as program directors and school superintendents who need to review aggregate reports on children's progress; users who are Reviewers have the ability to generate reports but cannot edit child records.

Within each role, you can assign certain permissions to each user. For example, you can ensure that a user who is a Provider has permission to access only the child records for the children with whom he or she works. As another example, you can enable users who are Reviewers to see "identified data" (data that includes identifying information such as children's names) or only "de-identified data" (data the system strips of all identifying information).

You can assign users to more than one role. This means that if you or someone else in your program is an Administrator who works directly with children, you can assign the roles of both Administrator **and** Provider.

This also means that you can allow a Provider in your program to run aggregate reports on all of the children, not just on those to whom he or she is assigned, by assigning the roles of both Provider and Reviewer.

> *Note: Anyone who is assigned the dual role of Provider and Reviewer will be able to see identifying data in the aggregate reports.*

Assigning the dual roles of Administrator and Reviewer has no practical purpose since an Administrator already has all of the capabilities allowed by the Reviewer role.

Manage Administrators

Depending on the size of your program, you may want to create additional Administrators to help you manage your AEPSi account. Administrators have the ability to perform the following actions:

- Create other users (Administrators, Reviewers, and Providers)
- Create child records
- Assign Providers (team members) to children
- Archive and delete child records
- Have access to all Child Reports, Class Reports, and Program Reports
- Export all data on any child in the program or all of the program's data

Creating a New Administrator

To create a new Administrator:

1. Click the *Manage Administrators* link on the left menu.

This will take you to the **Manage Administrators** page, where you will see a list of all of the Administrators currently in your program along with their names, titles, e-mail addresses, and phone numbers.

2. From the **Manage Administrators** page, click the *Create New Administrator* button.

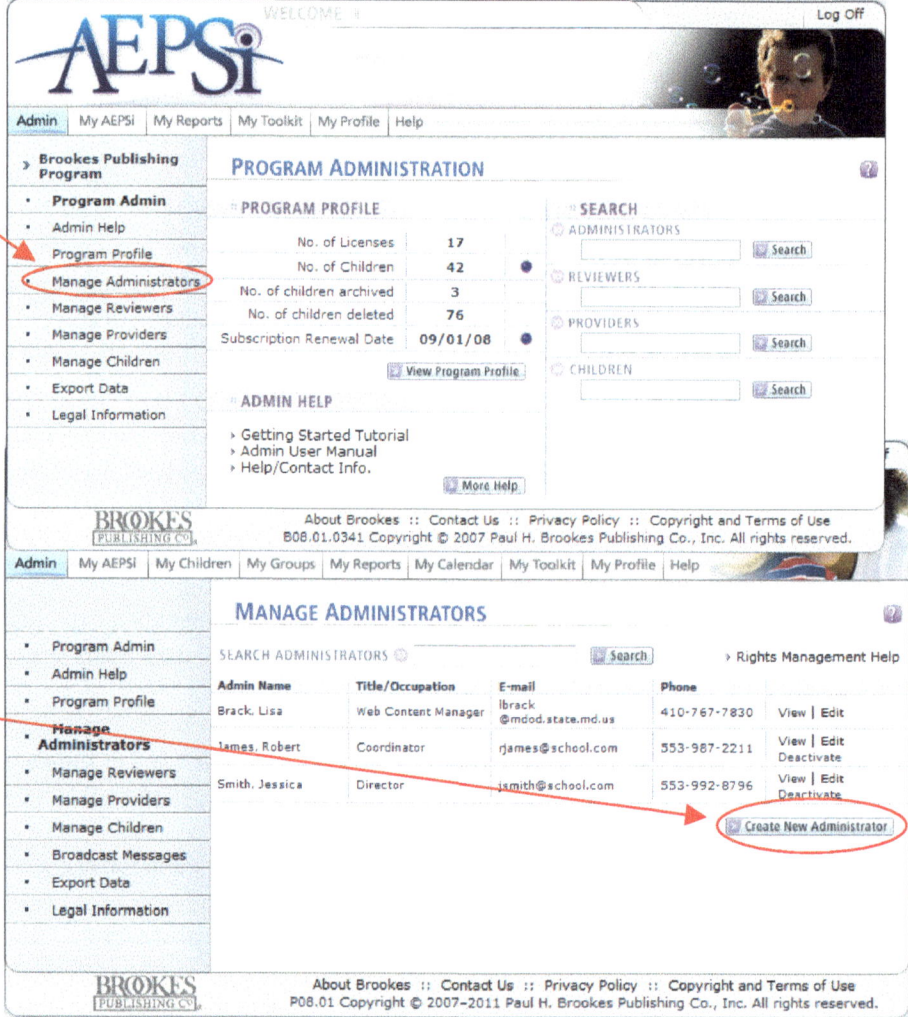

This will take you to the **Create Administrator** page, which is essentially a profile page for the user.

3. Since you accessed this page through the *Manage Administrators* link, the box next to Administrator will already be checked.

4. The Child Data Access permission is set to Yes by default. This means that the Administrator is able to run individual Child Reports, as well as Provider, Class, and Program Reports that include the child name. If that option is set to Yes, when generating reports, the Administrator also has the additional option to include or exclude the child's name. If the Administrator does not need to see child identifying information, set the Child Data Access option to No. An Administrator with no child data access only has access to Provider, Class, and Program Reports. The child name is replaced by X's.

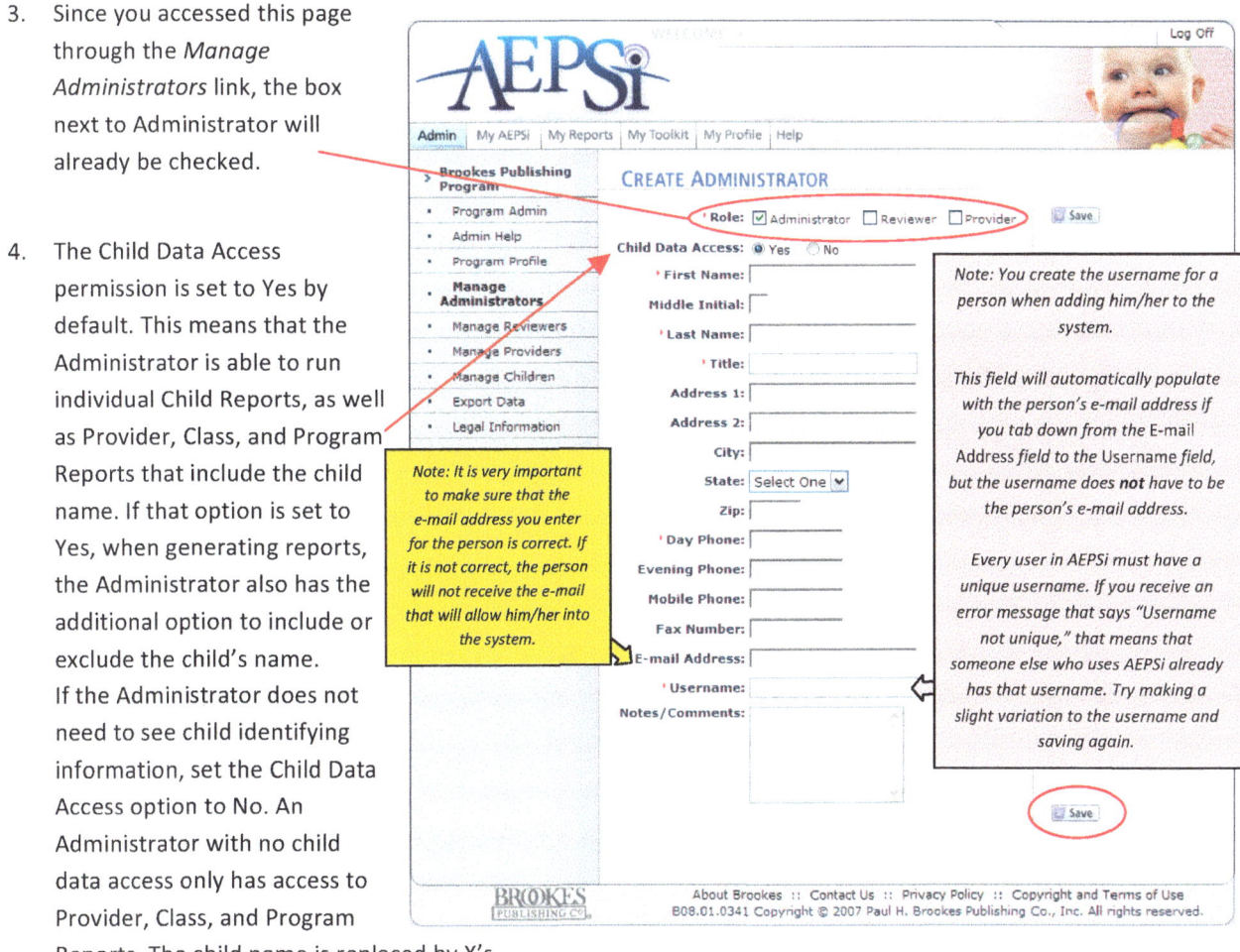

5. Enter the profile information for the Administrator. Items marked with a red arrow are required.

6. Once you have entered the profile information for the Administrator, click the *Save* button.

7. An e-mail will be sent to the Administrator that will contain a link to create his or her password. The Administrator will then be able to log in to the AEPSi account.

Note: If the Administrator does not receive an e-mail after being added to the system, there are two possible issues: 1) The e-mail address entered into his or her profile is incorrect—check to make sure it was entered properly, and 2) If the e-mail address was properly entered, inform the user to check his or her spam filter for the login e-mail.

Editing an Administrator Profile

If you need to edit a particular Administrator's profile, there are two options:

1. From your **Program Administration** main page, type the first or last name of the Administrator in the search field and click the *Search* button. The matching Administrator will show up in the search results. You can click the *Edit* link to make changes to the Administrator's profile. Once you have made the changes, click the *Save* button.
2. From your **Program Administration** main page, click the *Manage Administrators* link on the left menu. A list of all Administrators in your program will appear with links to view and edit their profiles.

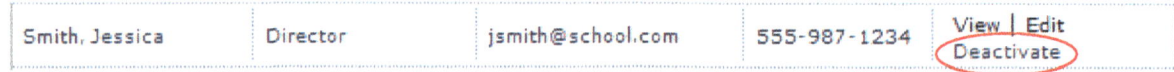

Deactivating/Reactivating/Deleting an Administrator

If an Administrator no longer needs access to his or her AEPSi account, you can deactivate the Administrator. To do this:

1. Click the *Manage Administrators* link on the left menu or use the Search function on the **Program Administration** page.
2. Locate the Administrator you would like to deactivate and click the *Deactivate* link.

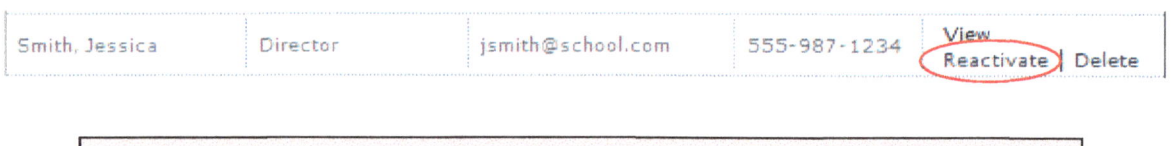

Once the Administrator has been deactivated, he or she will no longer be able to log into the AEPSi account. However, the Administrator's information will not be deleted and can be reactivated. If you need to reactivate an Administrator:

1. Click the *Manage Administrators* link on the left menu.
2. Locate the Administrator you would like to reactivate and click the *Reactivate* link.

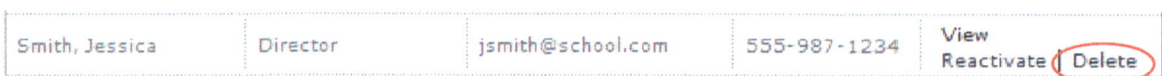

> *Note: You can only view, not edit, the profile of an Administrator who has been deactivated.*

To permanently remove a deactivated Administrator:

1. Click the *Manage Administrators* link on the left menu.
2. Locate the deactivated Administrator you would like to delete. All deactivated Administrators can be found at the bottom of your page.
3. Click the *Delete* link.

4. A confirmation message will display stating the following: "Are you sure you wish to delete this user? This action is permanent and cannot be undone."
5. Click *OK* to delete the user or *Cancel* if you do not wish to delete the user.

Once an Administrator has been deleted, all user account information will be permanently removed. The Administrator will no longer be able to access AEPSi.

> Note: Administrators must first be deactivated before they can be deleted.

Manage Reviewers

Another predefined role is Reviewer. A Reviewer will have access to Class and Program Reports. If you allow Reviewers access to identified child data, they will be able to view individual Child Reports in addition to the other reports. Reviewers will not be able to create or edit child records, or enter assessment data for children. Reviewers who do not have access to identified child data will not be able to view individual Child Reports and will not be able to see children's names on aggregate reports.

Creating a New Reviewer

To create a new Reviewer:

1. Click the *Manage Reviewers* link on the left menu.

This will take you to the **Manage Reviewers** page.

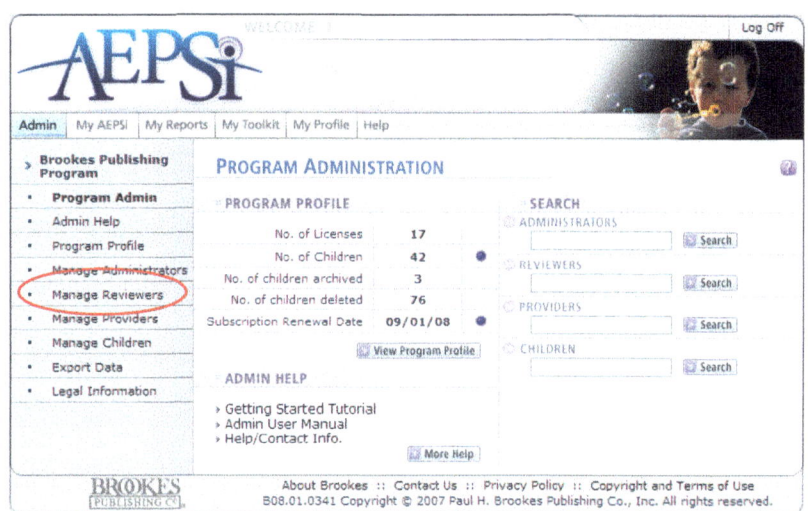

On the **Manage Reviewers** page you will see a list of all of the Reviewers currently in your program along with their names, titles, e-mail addresses, and phone numbers.

2. From the **Manage Reviewer** page, click the *Create New Reviewer* button.

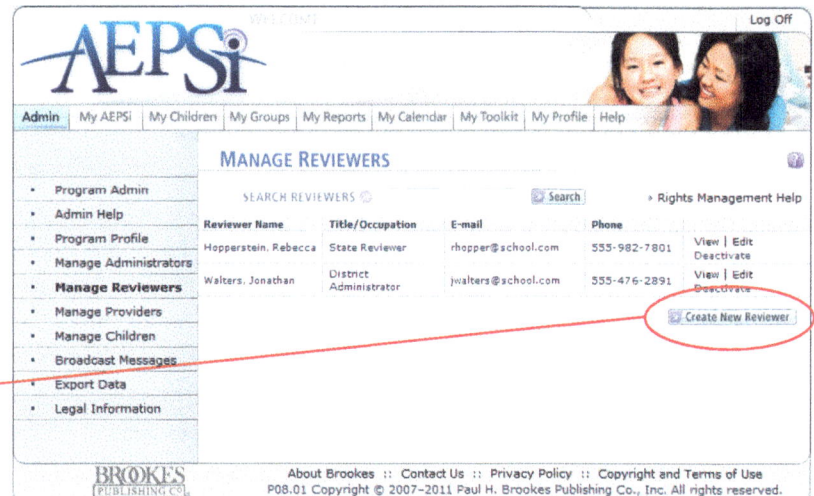

This will take you to the **Create Reviewer** page.

3. Since you accessed this page from the *Manage Reviewers* link, the box next to "Reviewer" will already be checked.

4. If the Reviewer should have access to identified child data, then click *Yes* for Child Data Access. Otherwise, click *No*.

5. Enter the profile information for the Reviewer. Items marked with a red arrow are required.

6. Once you have entered the profile information for the Reviewer, click the *Save* button.

7. An e-mail will be sent to the Reviewer that contains a link to create his or her password. The Reviewer will then be able to log in to the AEPSi account.

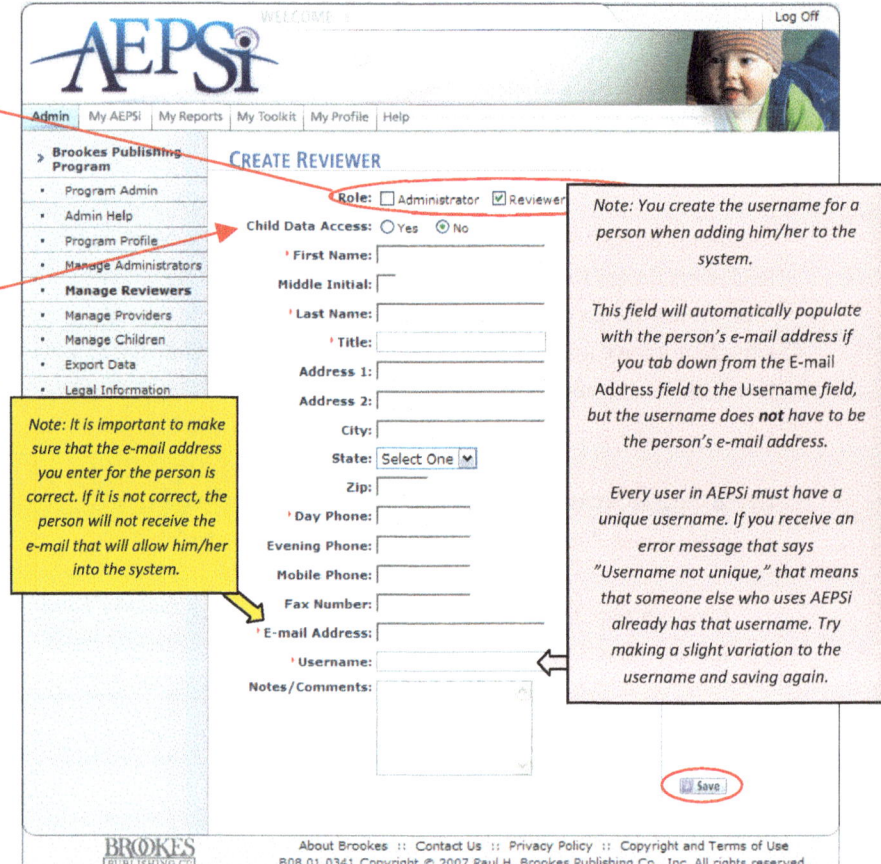

Note: If the Reviewer does not receive an e-mail after he or she has been created in the system, there are two possible issues:
1) The e-mail address entered into his or her profile is incorrect—check to make sure it was entered properly, and
2) If the e-mail address was properly entered, inform the user to check his or her spam filter for the login e-mail.

Editing a Reviewer Profile

If you need to edit a Reviewer's profile, there are two options:

1. From the **Program Administration** main page, type the first or last name of the Reviewer in the search field and click the *Search* button. The matching Reviewer will show up in the search results. You can click the *Edit* link to make changes to the Reviewer's profile.

2. From the **Program Administration** main page, you may also click the *Manage Reviewers* link on the left menu. A list of all Reviewers in your program will appear with links to view and edit their profiles.

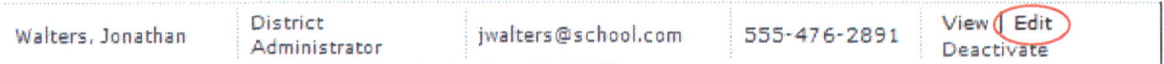

Deactivating/Reactivating/Deleting a Reviewer

If a Reviewer no longer needs access to the AEPSi account, you can deactivate that Reviewer. To do this:

12 | AEPSi Administrator Guide

1. Click the *Manage Reviewers* link on the left menu or use the search function on the **Program Administration** page.
2. Locate the Reviewer you would like to deactivate and click the *Deactivate* link.

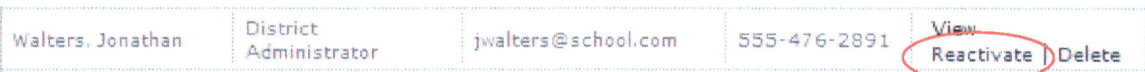

> Note: You can only view, not edit, the profile of a Reviewer who has been deactivated.

Once the Reviewer has been deactivated, he or she will no longer be able to log into the AEPSi account. However, the Reviewer's information will not be deleted and can be reactivated. If you need to reactivate a Reviewer:
1. Click the *Manage Reviewers* link on the left menu.
2. Locate the Reviewer you would like to reactivate and click the *Reactivate* link.

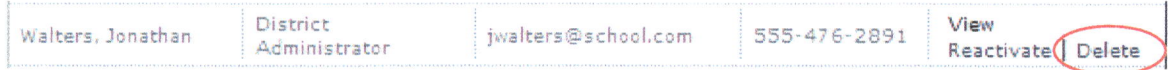

To permanently remove a deactivated Reviewer:
1. Click the *Manage Reviewers* link on the left menu.
2. Locate the deactivated Reviewer you would like to delete. All deactivated Reviewers can be found at the bottom of your **Manage Reviewers** page.
3. Click the *Delete* link next to the Reviewer you would like to delete.

4. A confirmation message will display stating the following: "Are you sure you wish to delete this user? This action is permanent and cannot be undone."
5. Click *OK* to delete the user or *Cancel* if you do not wish to delete the user.

Once a Reviewer has been deleted, all user account information will be permanently removed. The Reviewer will no longer be able to access AEPSi.

> Note: Reviewers must first be deactivated before they can be deleted.

Manage Providers

A Provider is any professional, employee, or contractor of your organization—such as teachers and therapists—who works directly with children. Providers have the ability to:
- Create/edit child records
- Enter child assessment data
- Create child journal entries
- Add/edit calendar events
- View, create, and export Child and Class reports

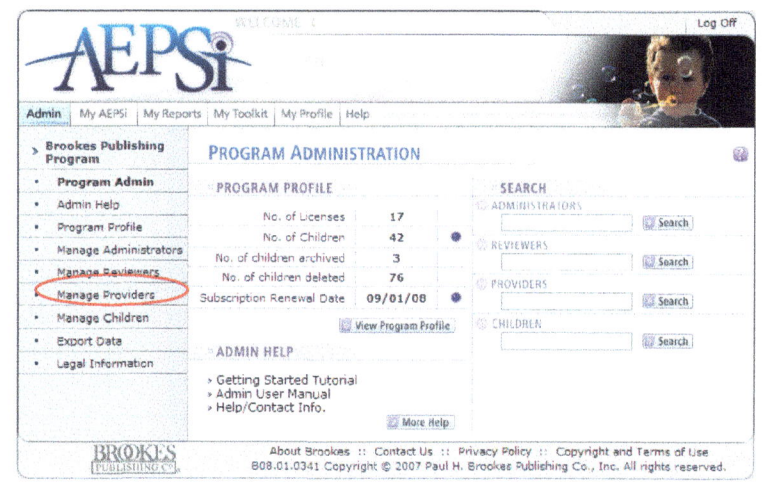

Creating a New Provider

To create a new Provider:

1. Click the *Manage Providers* link on the left menu. This will take you to the **Manage Providers** page, where you will see a list of all of the Providers currently in your system along with their names, titles, and e-mail addresses.

2. Click the *Create New Provider* button.

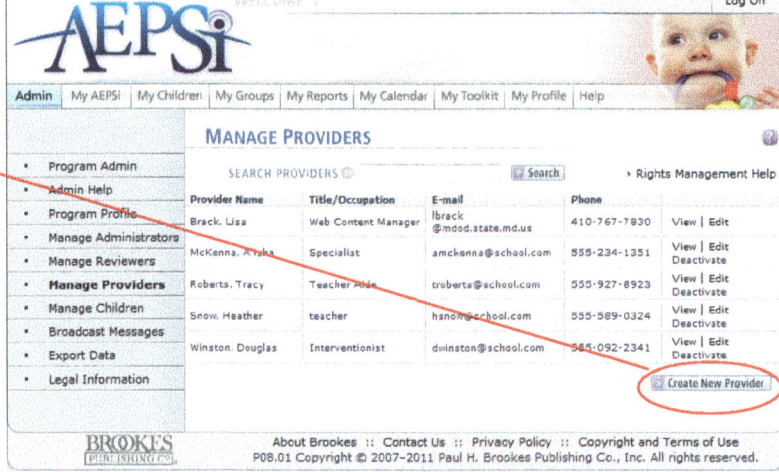

This will take you to the **Create Provider** page.

3. Since you accessed this page through the *Manage Administrators* link, the box next to Administrator will already be checked.

4. Enter the profile information for the Provider. On the profile page, required items are marked with a red arrow.

5. Once you have entered the profile information for the Provider, click the *Save* button.

6. An e-mail will be sent to the Provider that contains a link to create his or her password. The Provider will then be able to log in to the AEPSi account.

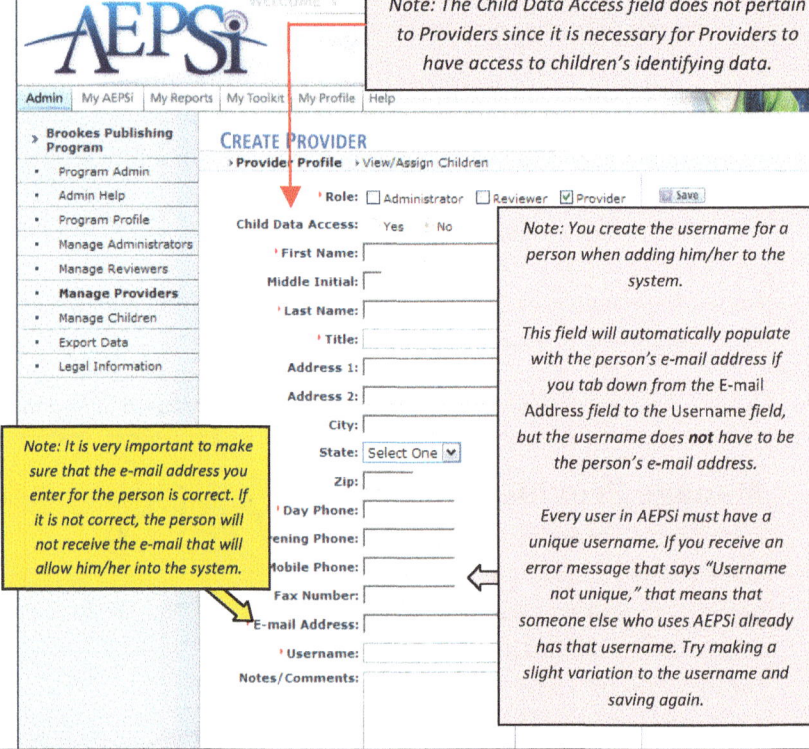

Note: The Child Data Access field does not pertain to Providers since it is necessary for Providers to have access to children's identifying data.

Note: You create the username for a person when adding him/her to the system.

*This field will automatically populate with the person's e-mail address if you tab down from the E-mail Address field to the Username field, but the username does **not** have to be the person's e-mail address.*

Every user in AEPSi must have a unique username. If you receive an error message that says "Username not unique," that means that someone else who uses AEPSi already has that username. Try making a slight variation to the username and saving again.

Note: It is very important to make sure that the e-mail address you enter for the person is correct. If it is not correct, the person will not receive the e-mail that will allow him/her into the system.

Note: If the Reviewer does not receive an e-mail after he or she has been created in the system, there are two possible issues:
1) The e-mail address entered into his or her profile is incorrect—check to make sure it was entered properly, and
2) If the e-mail address was properly entered, inform the user to check his or her spam filter for the login e-mail.

Editing a Provider Profile

If you need to edit a Provider's profile, there are two options:
1. From your **Program Administration** main page, type the name of the Provider in the search field box and click the *Search* button. The matching Provider will show up in the search results. You can click the *Edit* link to make changes to the Provider's profile.
2. From your **Program Administration** main page, you may also click the *Manage Providers* link on the left menu. A list of all Providers in your program will appear with links to view and edit their profiles.

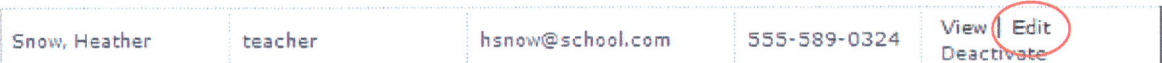

Deactivating/Reactivating/Deleting a Provider

If a Provider no longer needs access to the AEPSi account, you can deactivate that Provider. To do this:
1. Click the *Manage Providers* link on the left menu or use the search function on the **Program Administration** page.
2. Locate the Provider you would like to deactivate and click the *Deactivate* link.

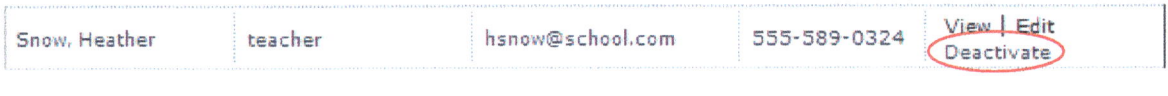

> Note: You are only able to view, not edit, the profile of a Provider who has been deactivated.

Once the Provider has been deactivated, he or she will no longer be able to log into the AEPSi account. However, the Provider's information will not be deleted and can be reactivated. Also, child records will retain all relevant provider information. If you need to reactivate a Provider:
1. Click the *Manage Providers* link on the left menu.
2. Locate the Provider you would like to reactivate and click the *Reactivate* link.

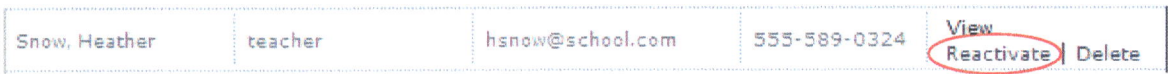

To permanently remove a deactivated Provider:
1. Click the *Manage Providers* link on the left menu.
2. Locate the deactivated Provider you would like to delete. All deactivated Providers can be found at the bottom of your **Manage Providers** page.
3. Click the *Delete* link.

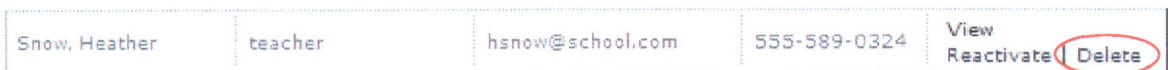

4. A confirmation message will display stating the following: "Are you sure you wish to delete this user? This action is permanent and cannot be undone."
5. Click *OK* to delete the user or *Cancel* if you do not wish to delete the user.

Once a Provider has been deleted, all user account information will be permanently removed. The Provider will no longer be able to access AEPSi.

> Note: A Provider must first be deactivated before he or she can be deleted.

Assigning Children to Providers

Once you have Providers and child records in your account (for information on creating child records, see **Section 3: Managing My Children**) you are able to assign children to Providers. Providers will only be able to access child records that have either been assigned to them or that they have created themselves.

To assign children to a Provider:

1. On the **Manage Provider** page, click the *Edit* link next to the Provider to whom you would like to assign children. This will take you to the profile page of that Provider.

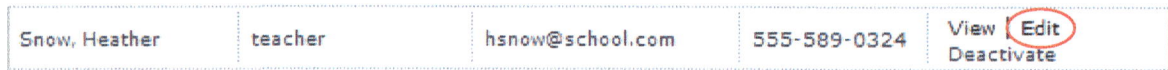

2. From the Provider's profile, click on the *View/Assign Children* link at the top of page.

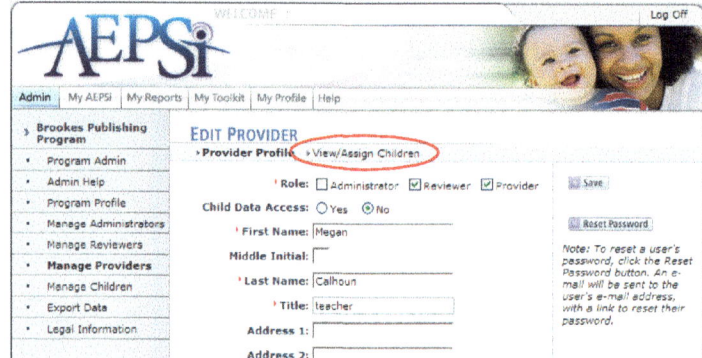

This will take you to the **Assign Children** page for that Provider, on which you will see a list of all of the children to whom that Provider is currently assigned. If there are no children listed, the Provider does not currently have any children assigned to him or her.

3. To assign children to the Provider, click the *Assign Additional Children* button.

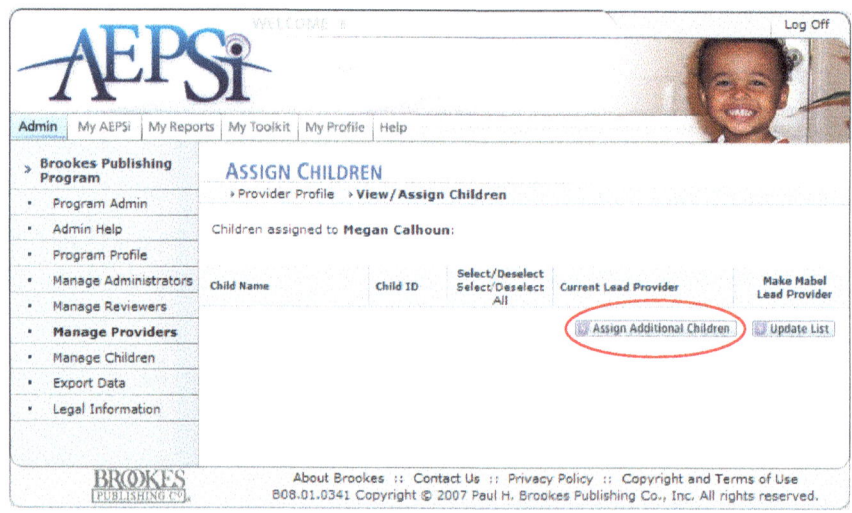

This will take you to the **Assign Children** page, where you will see a list of all the children who are in your program. If you have not created any child records, see **Section 3: Managing Your Children**.

4. To assign one or more children to the Provider, select the checkbox in the Select/Deselect column.

5. There is also an option to make the current Provider the Lead Provider for the selected child(ren). A Lead Provider has all of the rights and privileges of the Provider role but also can assign other Providers to a child's team. Each child can have one, and only one, Lead Provider.

6. Once you have selected the children and selected the Lead Provider options for the Provider, click the *Update List* button to save the information.

Removing Children Assigned to a Provider

To remove children assigned to a particular Provider:

1. Click the *Manage Providers* link on the left menu, and click the *Edit* link next to the Provider.
2. Click the *View/Assign Children* link at the top of the Provider's profile.
3. Deselect the child or children. Then click the *Update List* button.

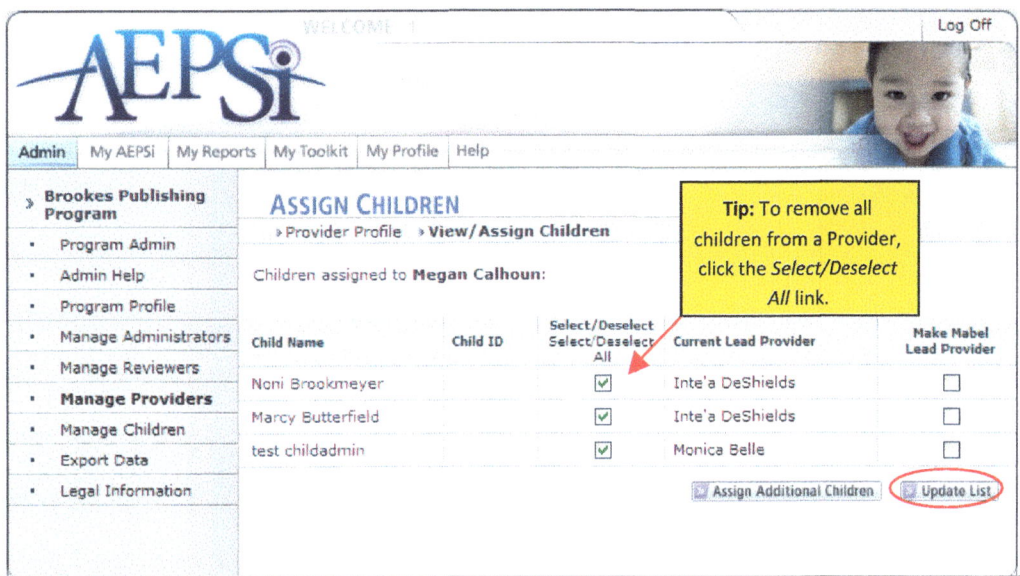

Note: Removing a child assigned to a Provider will not remove the child record from the AEPSi system. The Provider will simply no longer have access to the child profile and assessment data.

Assigning User Dual Roles

To assign a user to more than one role, simply check more than one box in the Role field when creating or editing a user's profile.

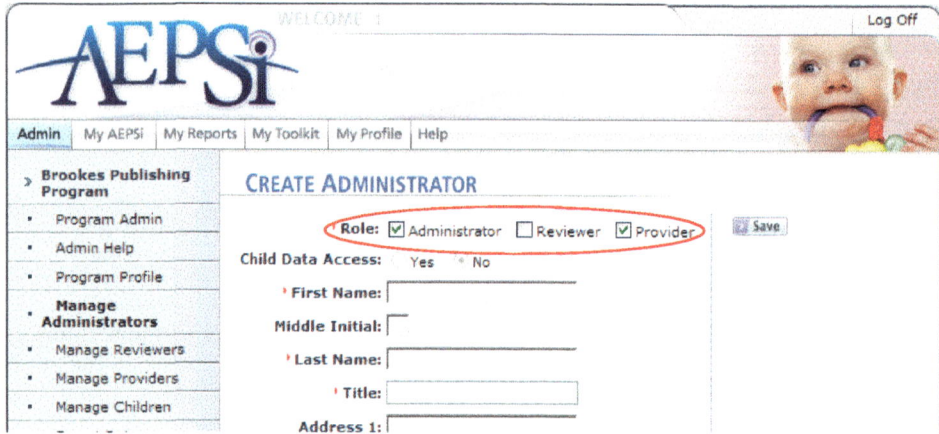

When assigning users with dual roles there are two options:

Administrator/Provider
- Has access to the **Admin** tab and is able to create new users and control their rights and access
- Can assign/reassign children to any Provider
- Is able to run Program Reports in addition to Child and Class Reports
- Can create new child records and enter any data pertaining to children (assessments, journal entries, calendar events, Family Reports, etc.)

Provider/Reviewer
- Can create new child records and enter any data pertaining to children (assessments, journal entries, calendar events, Family Reports, etc.)
- Is able to run Program Reports in addition to Child and Class Reports

Managing Your Children

Section 3

The following section describes how to create, edit, archive, and delete child records as well as how to assign Providers to a child's team.

Creating a Child Record

To create a child record:

1. Click the *Manage Children* link on the left menu.

   This will take you to the **Manage Children** page, where you will see a list of all of the children currently in your program along with their names and child IDs.

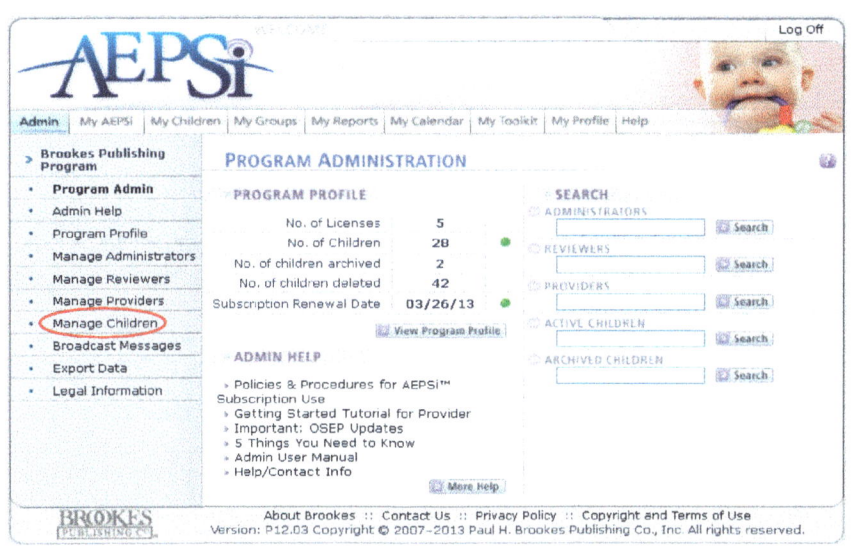

2. From the **Manage Children** page, click the *Create New Child Record* button.

   This will take you to the **Create Child Record** page, which is essentially a new child's profile page.

AEPSi Administrator Guide | 19

3. Enter the information on the child profile. Items marked with a red arrow are required.

4. In order for a child to be included in OSEP reporting, there are four required fields that must be completed:

   o Include in OSEP Reporting: Select *Yes* if the child will be included in OSEP reporting. If the child will not be included in OSEP reporting, select *No* and leave the funding source, program entry date, and program exit date at their default values.

   o Funding Source: Select whether the child is Early Childhood Sp Ed - Part B (3-5) or Early Intervention-Part C (Birth-3).

   o Program Entry Date: The date the child began receiving services.

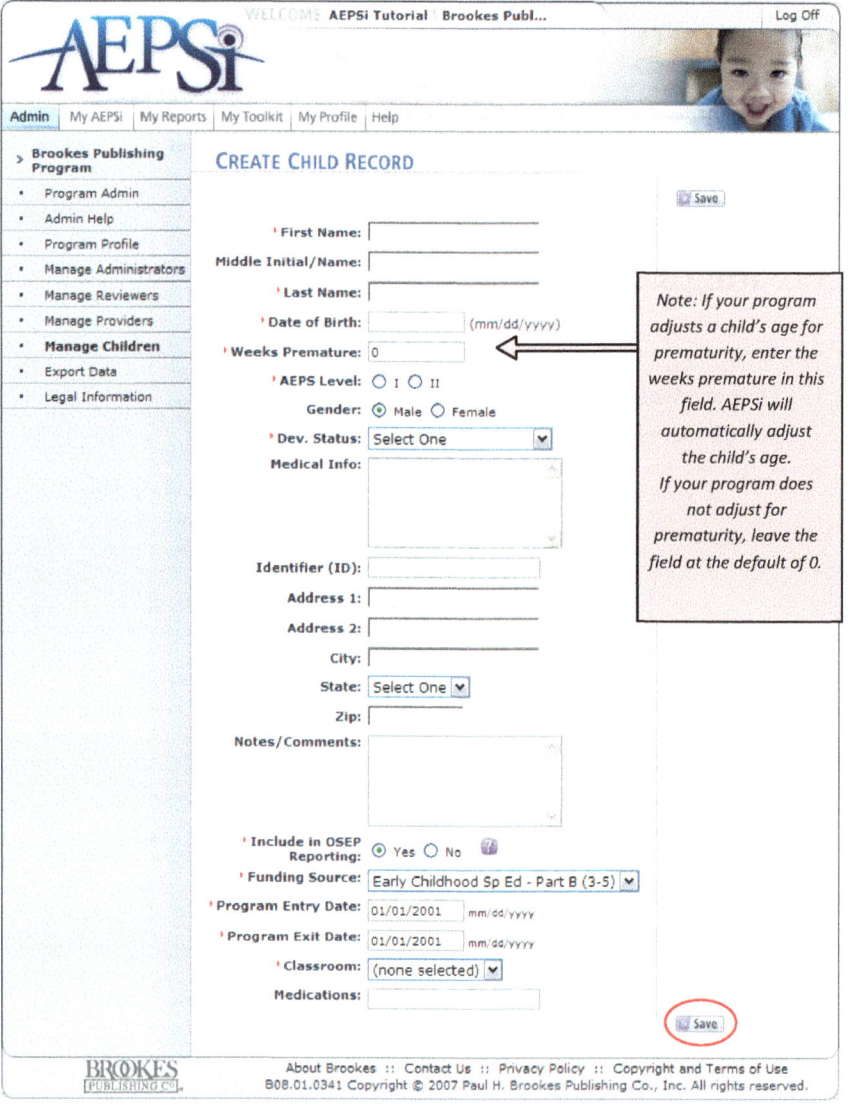

   o Program Exit Date: The date the child stopped receiving services. (*Note: Until you know the exit date for a child, you may leave the field at the default of 01/01/2001.*)

5. Once the required fields are entered for the child profile, click the *Save* button.

Custom Fields

As an Administrator, you have the ability to create custom fields that will be displayed on the **Child Profile** page. If there is any information that you would like to track in AEPSi (e.g., Social Security number, race/ethnicity), you can use the custom field feature. Five types of custom fields can be created: a text field, a number field, a date field, a yes/no field, or a dropdown menu. You also have the ability to specify whether or not a custom field is required and can select preformatted options for the custom fields.

Creating Custom Fields

To create a custom field:

Go to your **Admin Program Profile** on the left menu or select the *View Program Profile* button on the main Program Admin page.

Select the *Custom Fields* button.

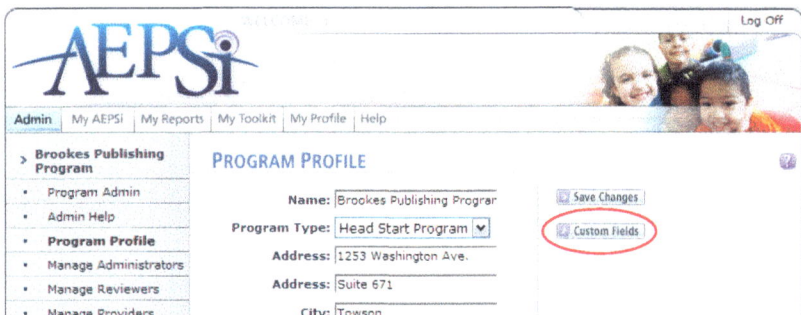

This will take you to the **Custom Fields** page, which will show a list of your current custom fields and allow you to create new custom fields.

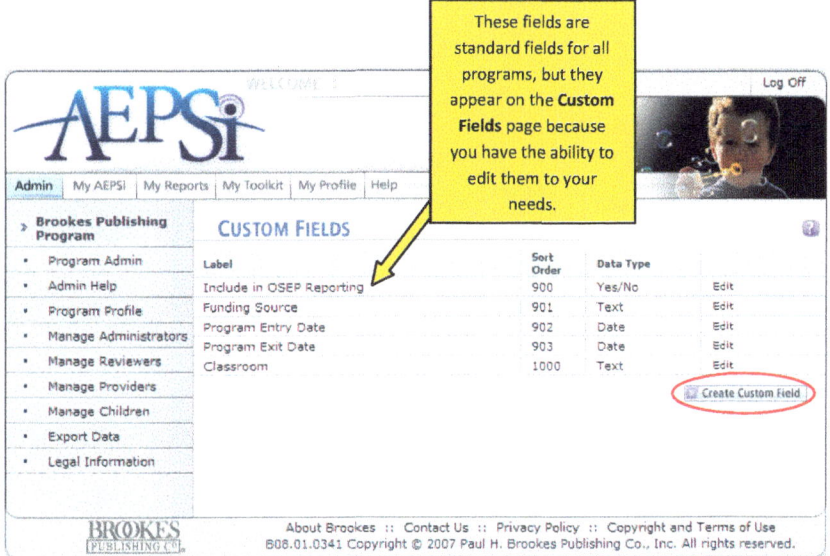

Select the *Create Custom Field* button.

This will take you to the **Edit Custom Field** page, where you will set up your custom field.

Custom Field Options

Below is a brief description of the custom field options that are available. Fields marked with an arrow are required.

- Label: Create a label for the custom field. The label is the name you would like your custom field to appear as on the **Child Profile** page.

- Sort Order: You can type in a number that will determine the order the custom fields will appear on the **Child Profile** page. The lower the number, the earlier in the order the field will appear. As a default, the number 1000 will appear when you create a new custom field. If all custom fields are left with this default value, the custom fields will appear in alphabetical order.

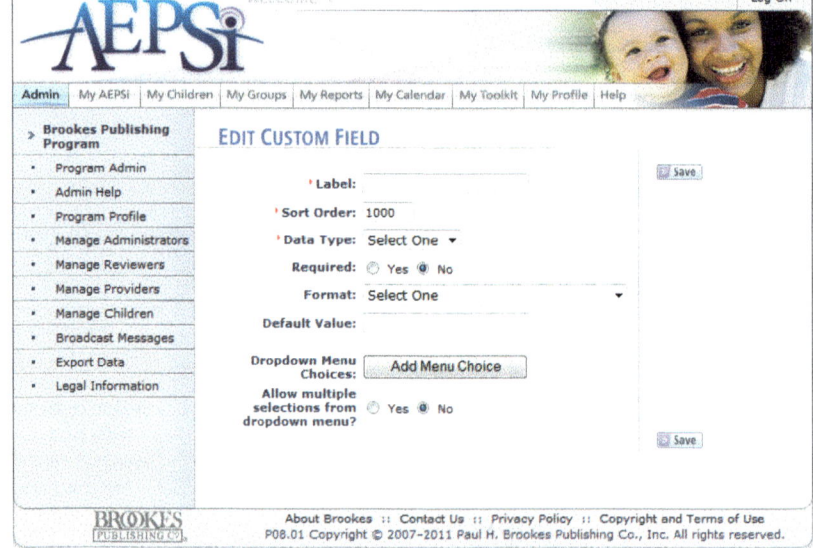

- Data Type: Select the type of custom field. The choices are text, number, date, or yes/no. If you are creating a dropdown menu, you must select text as the data type.

  Text: Field that holds any combination of numbers, letters, or characters.
  Number: Field that holds numbers only.
  Date: Field that holds a date in the format mm/dd/yyyy or mm/dd/yy.
  Yes/No: Field where user has the option to select either yes or no.

- Required: Here, you can specify whether you want the custom field to be required.

- Format: You can optionally select a format for the custom field. Options include Social Security number (999-99-9999), short date (mm/dd/yy), extended zip code (99999-9999), etc. Selecting a format for a custom field will require the user completing the field to enter the data in that format and no other. This can help maintain data accuracy.

- Default Value: You can optionally enter a default value for your custom field. When a user adds a new child profile, the default values will appear automatically in the custom field.

- Dropdown Menu Choices: If you want to create a dropdown menu for a text field, enter the choices you want to appear in the dropdown menu here.

- Allow multiple selections from dropdown menu?: This option only applies to the dropdown menu custom field. Selecting yes will allow users to select multiple choices from the dropdown menu by holding down the Ctrl key on the keyboard.

Once you have made your selections, click the *Save* button. The custom field will now appear on the **Child Profile** page for all children in your account.

To give you a better idea of how the custom fields work, the following section outlines creating each of the five types of fields: text field, number field, date field, yes/no field, and dropdown menu field.

Creating a Text Custom Field

To demonstrate this type of field, let's imagine that you would like to create a field on the child's profile for a Provider to record the medications a child is taking.

You decide to call this field "Medications," so this is what you enter into the *Label* field.

Since there is no particular order you want this field to appear in on the child's profile page, leave the sort order at the default of 1000.

For *Data Type,* select Text since this is a field that people will be able to write in.

This should not be a required field on the child's profile, so mark the Required field No.

There is no particular format for this field, so leave that blank.

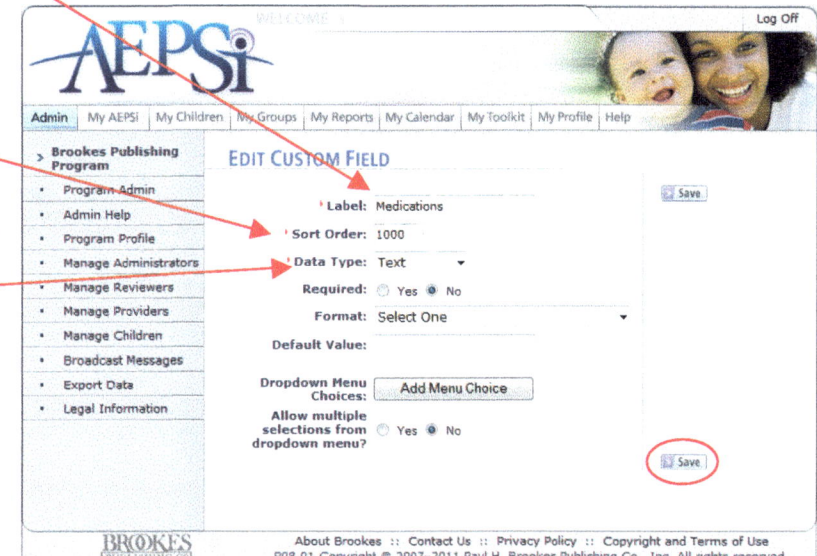

There are no default values or dropdown menu choices since this will not be a dropdown menu field, and you can skip the multiple selections option, which is only pertinent to dropdown menu fields.

Then click the *Save* button.

Your new custom field will now appear on the **Custom Fields** page.

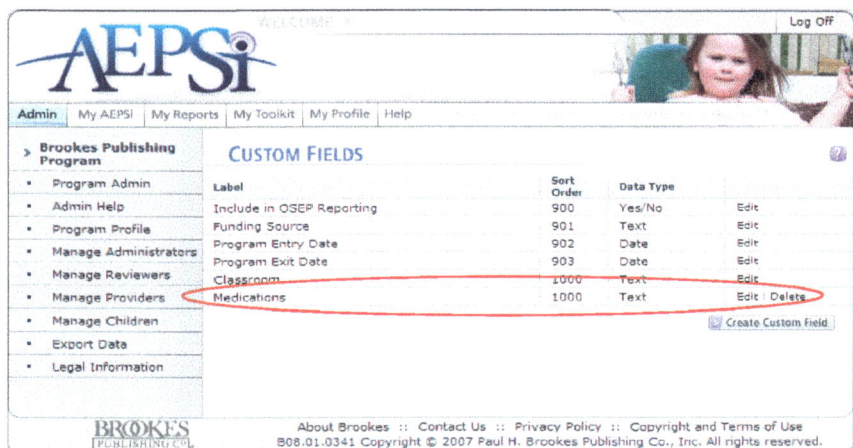

AEPSi Administrator Guide | 23

Creating a Number Custom Field

To demonstrate this type of field, let's imagine that you would like to create a field on the child's profile in which to enter the child's Social Security number.

Name this field "Social Security."

Leave the sort order at 1000.

Select Number for the Data Type since this field is a number.

Click Yes to make the field a required field on the child's profile.

Select the Social Security Number format from the *Format*

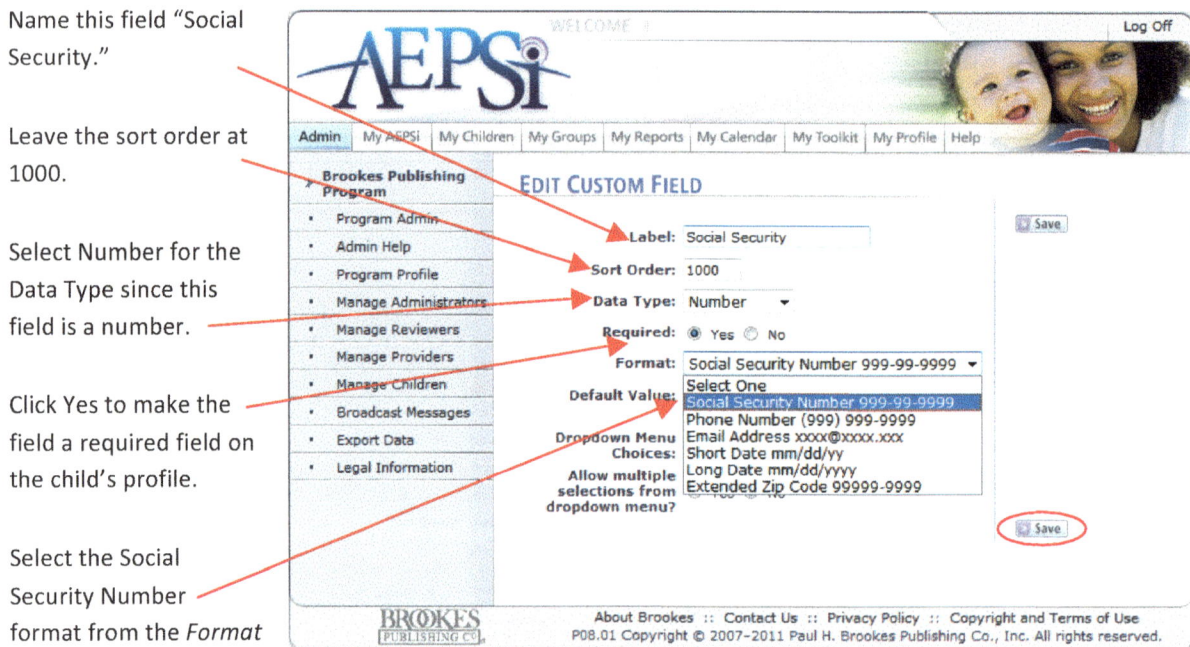

dropdown menu—this will ensure that users enter the Social Security number properly.

There is no default value for this field, so skip this item. Also skip items dealing with dropdown menus since this is a number field.

Then click the *Save* button.

Your new custom field now appears on the **Custom Fields** page.

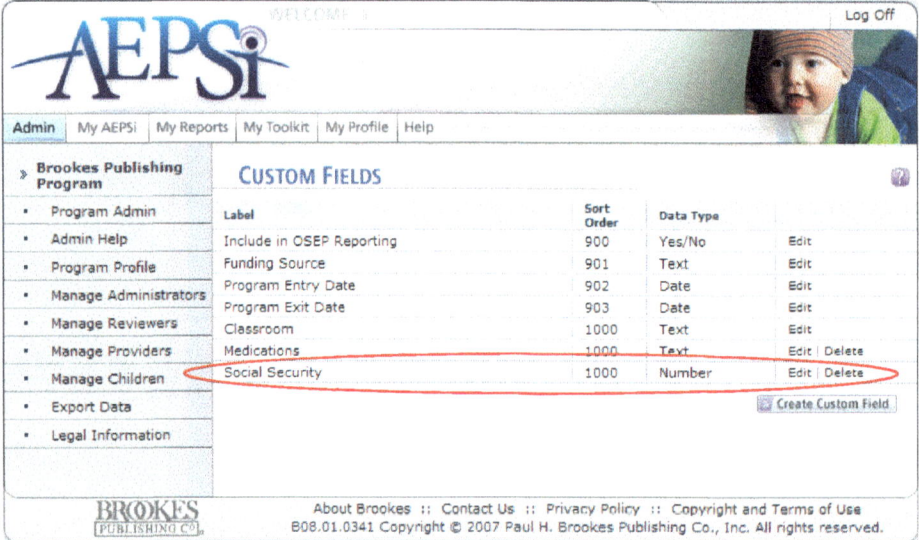

Creating a Date Custom Field

To demonstrate this type of field, let's imagine that your program would like a field on the child's profile in which to enter the date of the child's first IEP.

You decide to call this field "Initial IEP Date."

Leave the Sort Order at the default of 1000.

Select Date for Data Type.

Click No so that the field is not required on the child's profile.

For Format, select the Long Date so that users enter all four digits of the year.

There is no default value for this field since it is a date field, so skip the items dealing with dropdown menus.

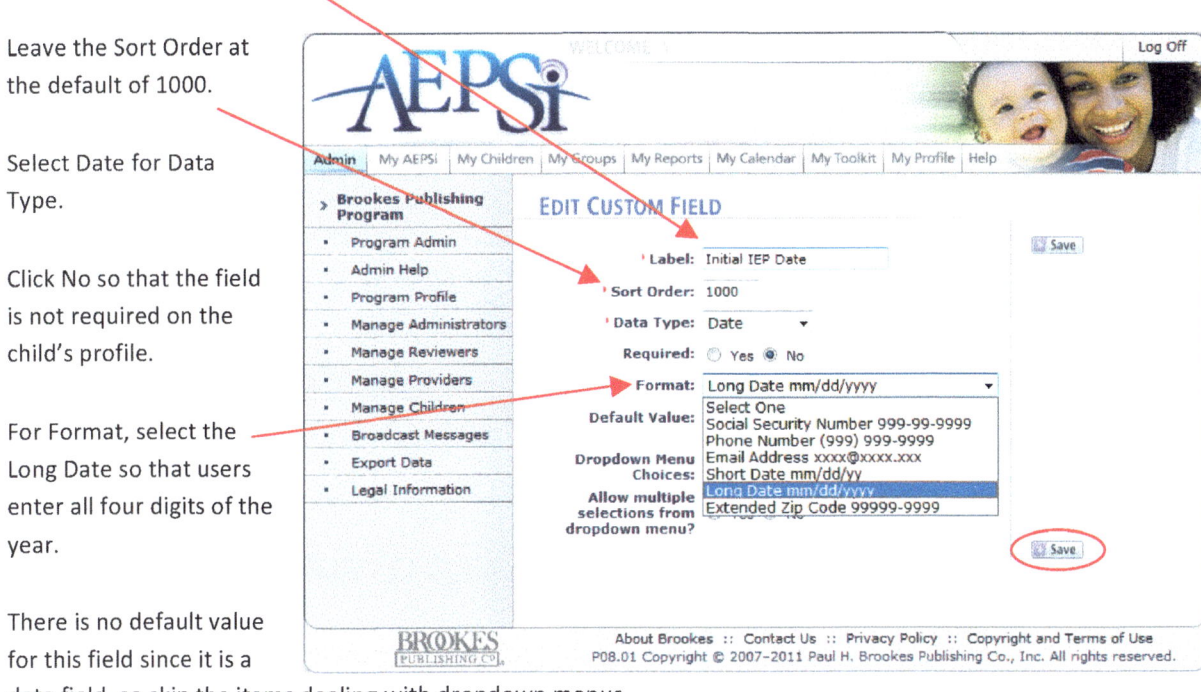

Then click the *Save* button.

Your new custom field now appears on the **Custom Fields** page.

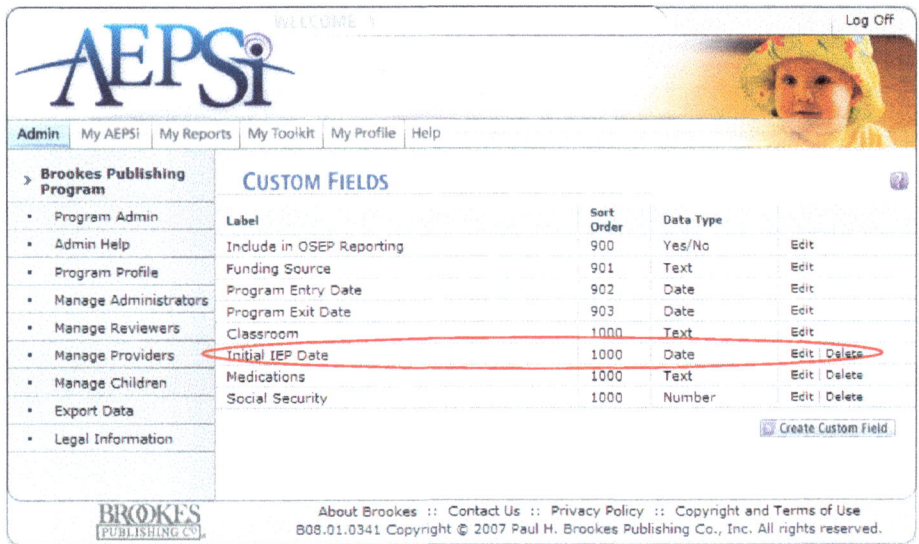

Creating a Yes/No Custom Field

To demonstrate this Custom type of field, let's imagine that you would like to create a field on the child's profile in which to capture whether the child has an IEP.

You want to call this field "Does child have an IEP?"

Since you want this field to appear before your Initial IEP Date field, make the sort order 999.

The data type of this field is Yes/No.

Because this information is important for your program to know, select Yes to make this a required field on the child's profile.

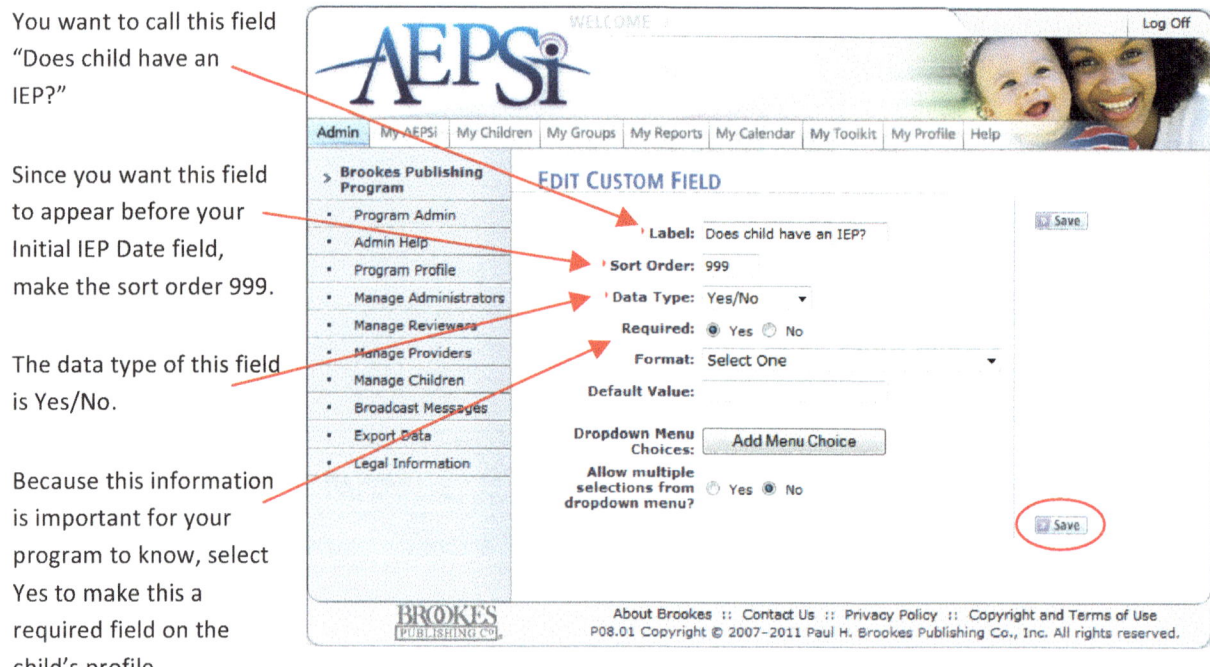

This field does not have a specific format, default value, or dropdown menu items, so skip these items.

You can now click the *Save* button.

Your new custom field now appears on the **Custom Fields** page, right above Initial IEP Date.

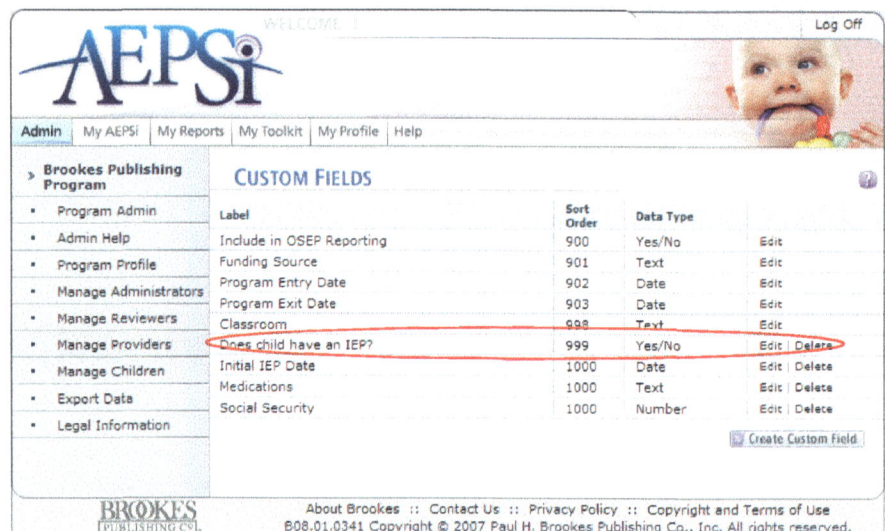

Creating a Dropdown Menu Custom Field

To demonstrate this type of field, let's imagine that you would like to create a field on the child's profile in which to capture the child's race/ethnicity.

Call this field "Race/Ethnicity" to match what is used on your program's intake forms.

Leave the sort order at the default of 1000.

The Data Type for this field is Text.

Click No so that the field is not required on the child's profile.

There is no specific format for this field, so skip this item.

Enter the choices you would like to appear in your dropdown menu in the Dropdown Menu Choices field.

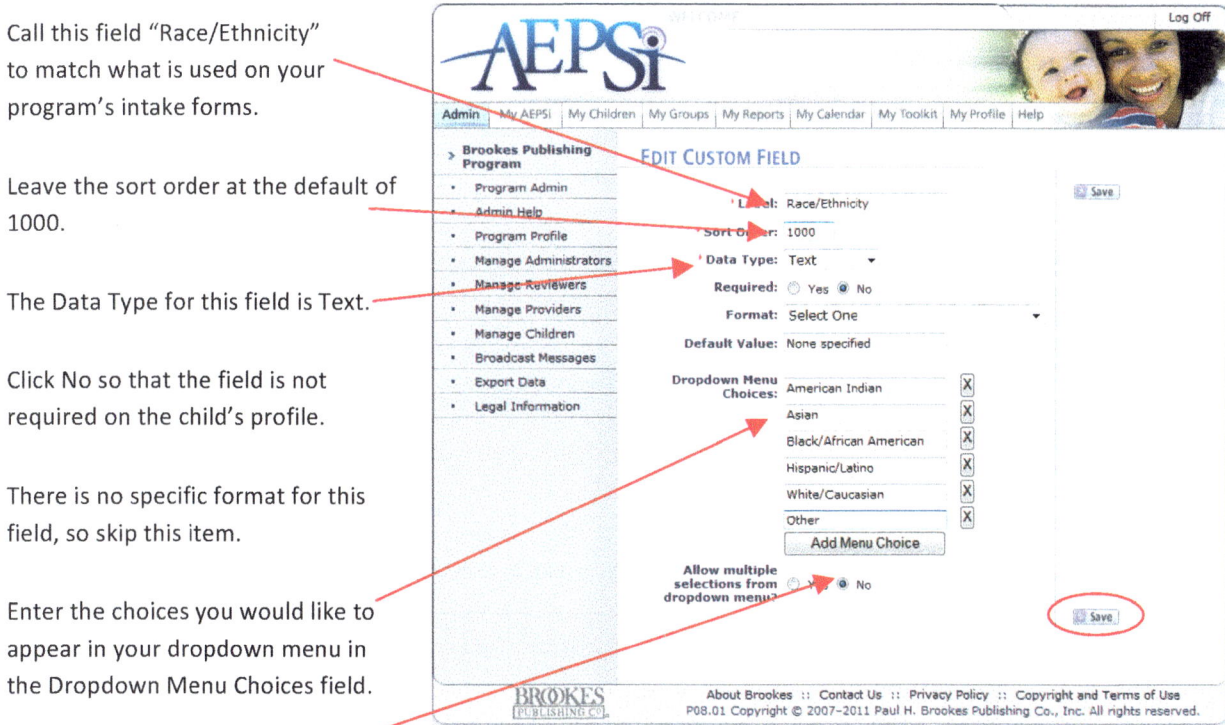

Select *No* to prevent users from selecting multiple options from the dropdown menu.

You can now click the *Save* button.

Your new custom field now appears on the **Custom Fields** page.

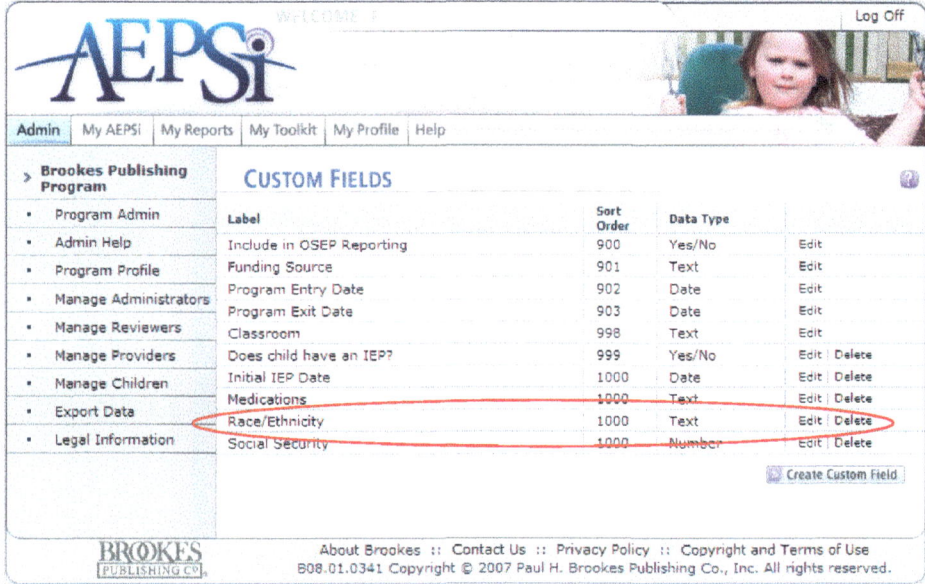

Now when you look at a child's profile, you will see all of the custom fields you created at the bottom of the profile page—and you will have the key data your program needs.

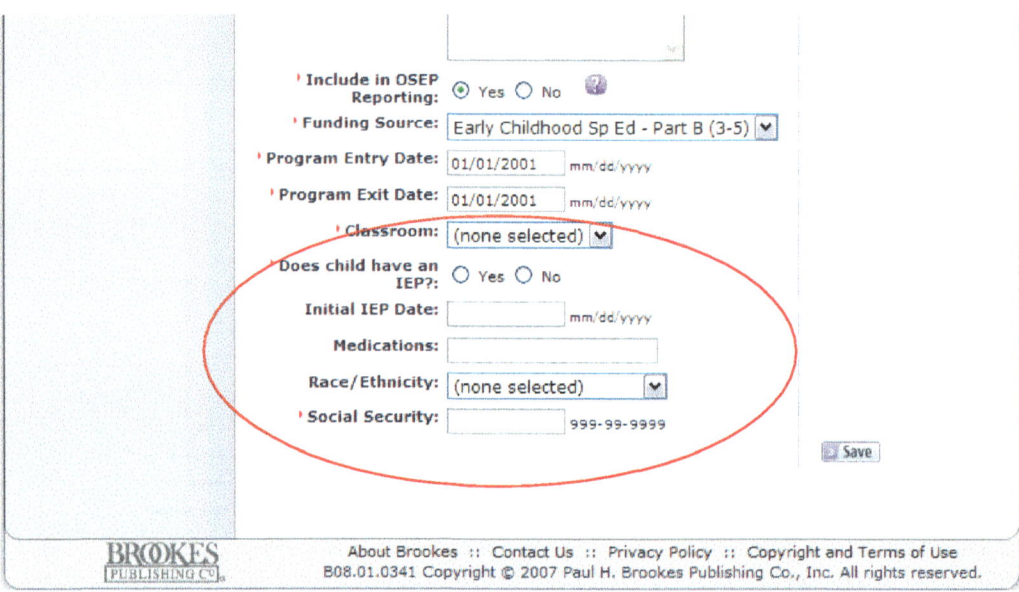

Edit/Delete a Custom Field

To edit or delete a custom field, select **Program Profile** from the left menu and click the *Custom Fields* button. Then select the *Edit* link to edit the custom field or the *Delete* link to delete the custom field.

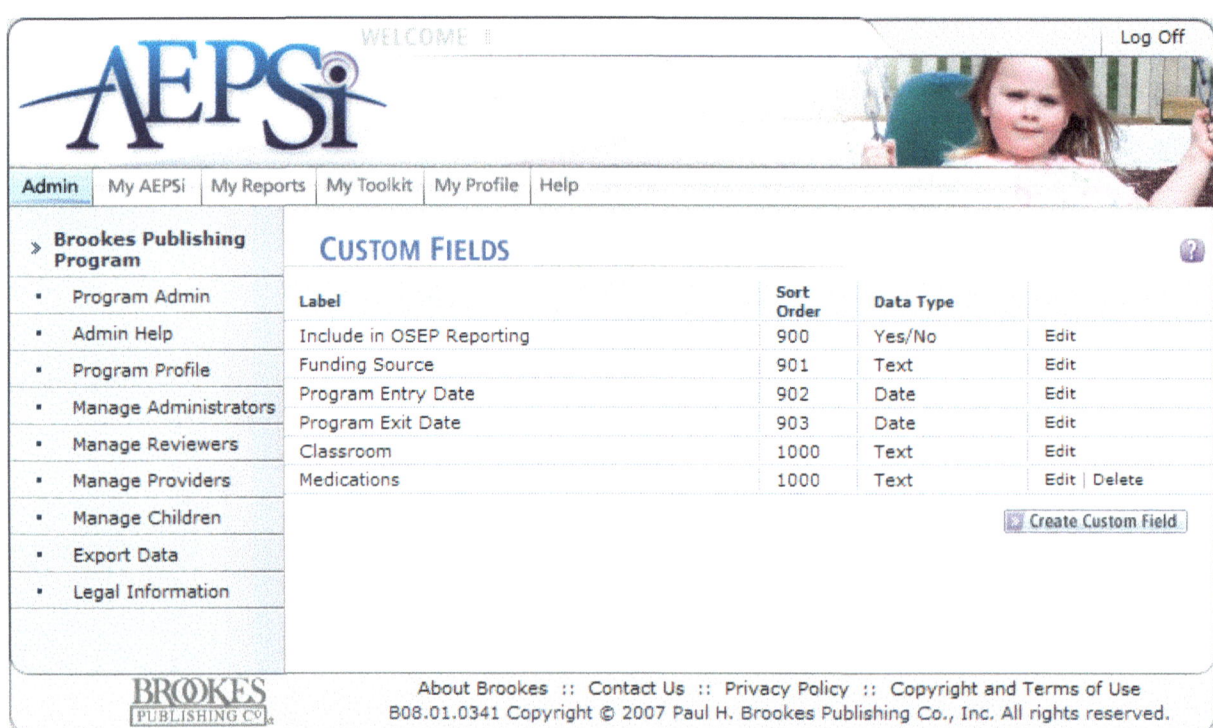

Note: The OSEP fields and the "Classroom" custom field cannot be deleted, and the label cannot be changed through the Edit *link.*

Note: If you are a part of an Enterprise account, your Enterprise has the ability to create custom fields for all programs under the Enterprise.

Updating a Child's Team

A child's team consists of the child's Caregiver(s) and the Providers who work directly with the child. These Providers will be able to enter assessment data for the child, create child journal entries, create calendar events relating to that specific child (which will be accessible by the entire team), create group assessment activities, and run various Child Reports.

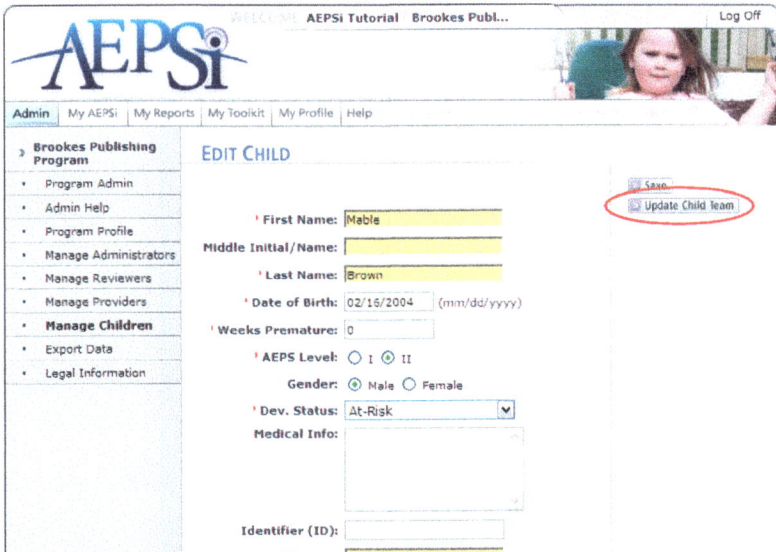

To add people to a child's team, go to the **Manage Children** page from the left menu navigation and select the *Edit* link next to the name of the child whose team you would like to update. Then select the *Update Child Team* button on the child's profile page.

This will take you to the **Update Child Team** page, where you will see a list of all of the providers in your program.

Assigning Providers to Children

Select the checkbox next to each Provider you would like to assign to the child. If no Providers appear in the list, see **Section 2: Managing Users** to learn how to create Provider records.

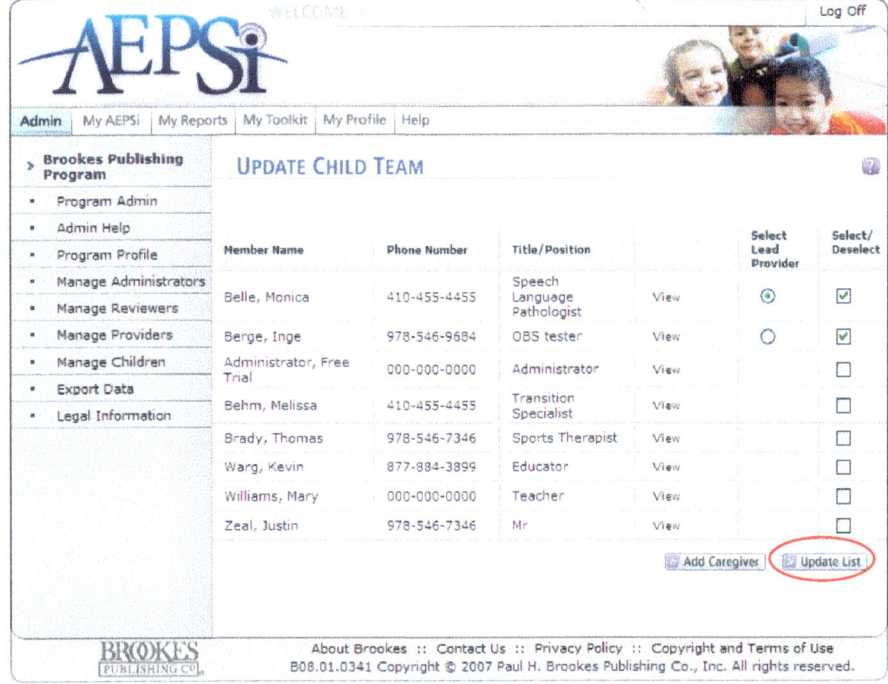

Next to the Select/Deselect column, there is a column called Select Lead Provider. In addition to the rights and privileges assigned to the Provider role, the Lead Provider has the ability to assign and remove other Providers from the child's team, add/edit Caregiver information, and designate another Lead Provider for a child.

Once all team members have been selected for the child, click the *Update List* button.

> *Note: If a Provider creates a child record in the system, he or she will automatically be that child's Lead Provider.*

Removing Providers from a Child's Team

Deselect the checkboxes of the Providers you would like to remove from the **Update Child Team** page and click the *Update List* button.

Remember that removing Providers from a child's team does **not** remove the users from your AEPSi account. The Provider will simply no longer be a member of that child's team or be able to view or edit that child's data.

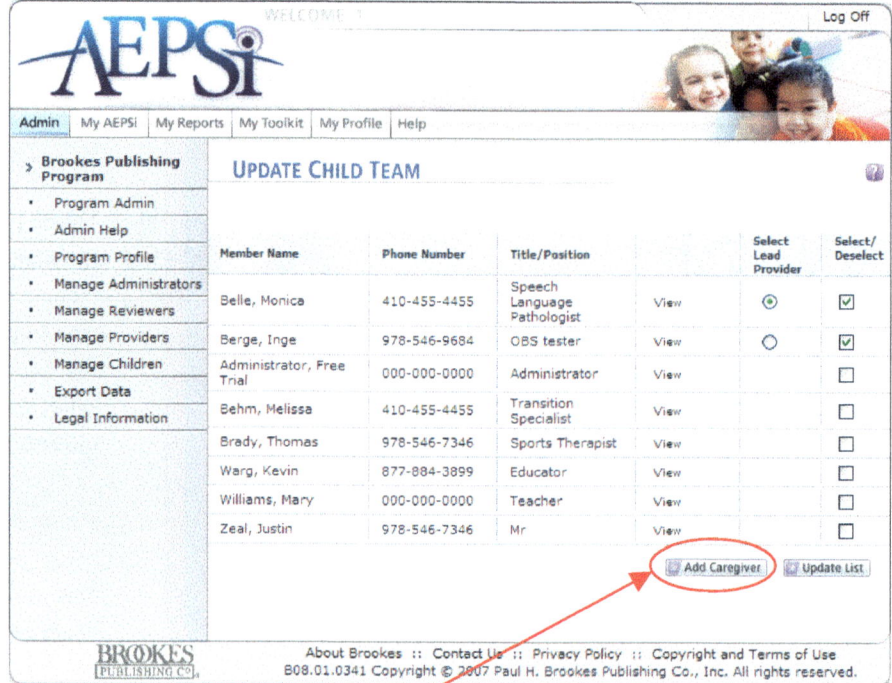

Creating a Caregiver Profile

To create a Caregiver for the child, click the *Add Caregiver* button at the bottom of the **Update Child Team** page.

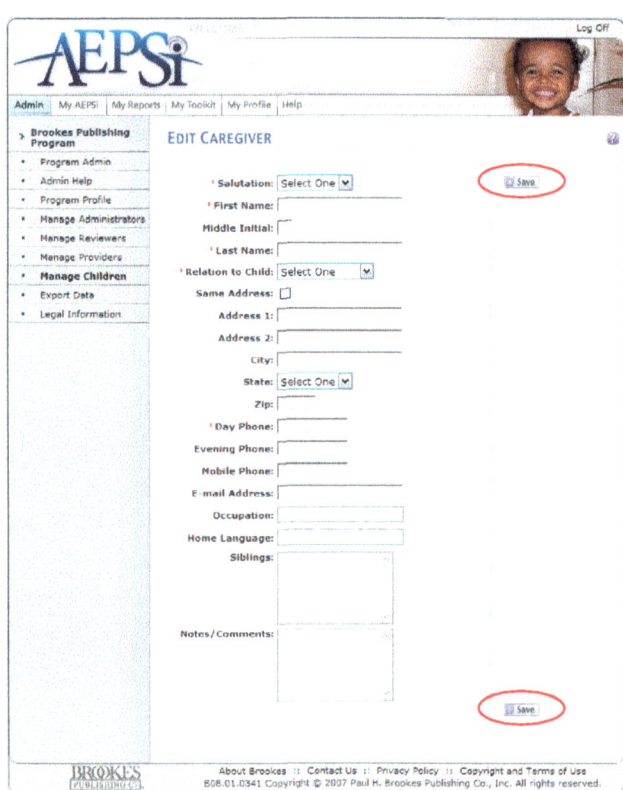

This will take you to the Caregiver profile page.

From here you can enter the Caregiver's profile information in the fields. Mandatory fields are designated with a red arrow.

Once you have completed entering the information, click the *Save* button.

Edit/Delete Caregiver Profile

To edit a Caregiver Profile, click the *Edit* link next to the Caregiver's name on the **Update Child Team** page.

Make changes to the Caregiver Profile and then click the *Save* button.

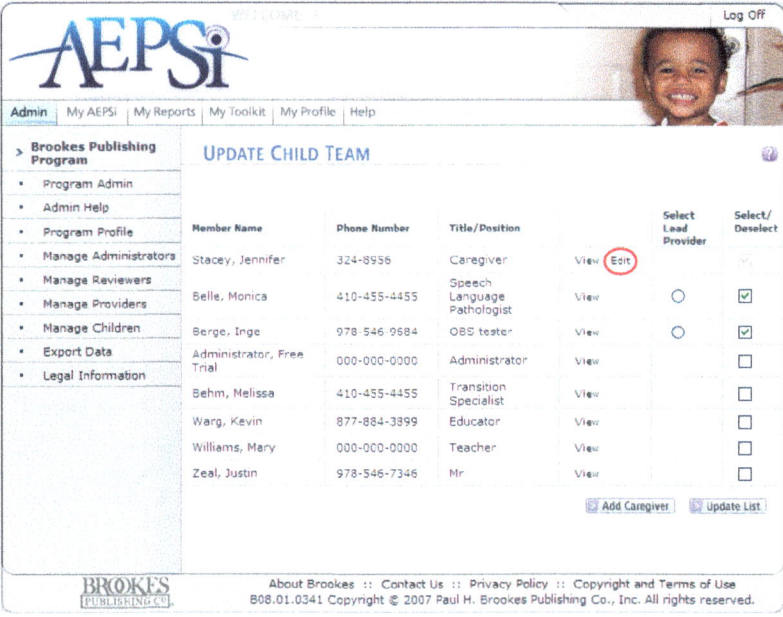

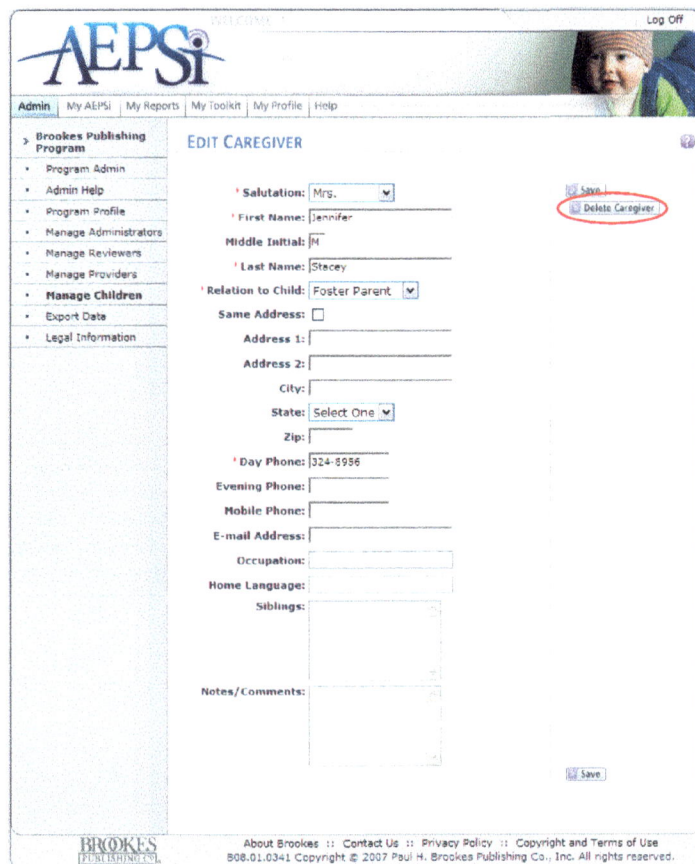

To delete a Caregiver, click the *Edit* link next to the Caregiver's name on the **Update Child Team** page.

When it takes you to the child's profile, click the *Delete Caregiver* button.

Archiving/Deleting a Child Record

Once a child no longer needs an active record (e.g., the child has moved, the child has aged out of the program), there are two options: *archiving* the child record or *deleting* the child record.

Archiving a child record means Providers will no longer be able to create, edit, or view assessments, journal entries, or individual Child Reports, and the child's profile will no longer be open to editing. However, all information relating to a child record will remain in the system and can be viewed and included in class and program aggregate reports (including OSEP reports).

When a child record is deleted, all assessment data, reports, journal entries, and so forth will be permanently removed from the system and the child's data will not be included in any reports. It is recommended that *before* deleting a child record, you export that child's data. (See **Section 6**: **Exporting Data**.)

Archiving a Child Record

To archive a child record, go to the Active Children section of your **Manage Children** page and check the boxes next to the child or children you would like to archive under the Archive column. You can use the *Select/Deselect All* link to select all child records. Then click on the *Update List* button.

The child record(s) you have archived will now appear on the Archived Children section of the **Manage Children** page.

Reactivating an Archived Child Record

To reactivate an archived child record, select the *Archived Children* link on the **Manage Children** page. Either locate the child's name on the list of children, or use the Search function at the top of the page. Check the box(es) next to the child or children you would like to reactivate under the Reactivate column. You can also use the *Select/Deselect All* link to select all child records.

Click the *Update List* button.

The child records you reactivated will now appear on the Active Children section of the **Manage Children** page.

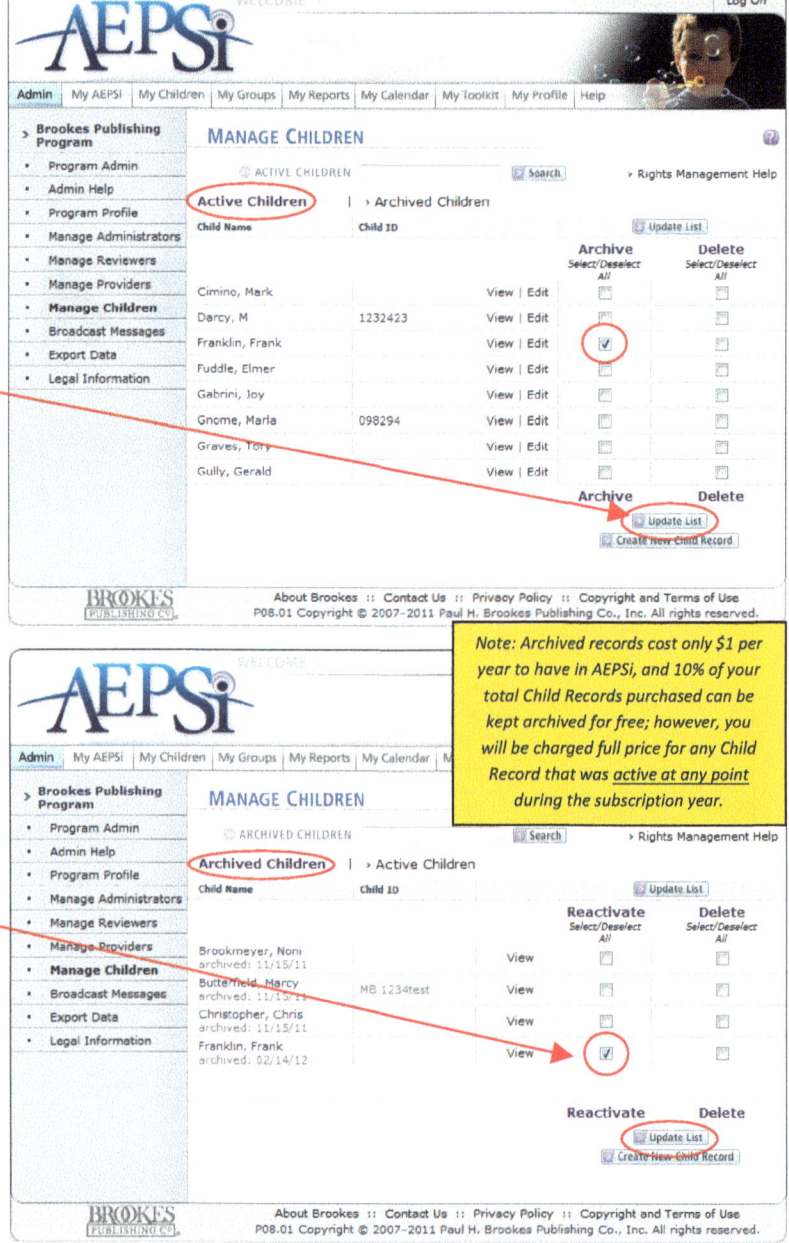

Note: Archived records cost only $1 per year to have in AEPSi, and 10% of your total Child Records purchased can be kept archived for free; however, you will be charged full price for any Child Record that was active at any point during the subscription year.

Deleting a Child Record

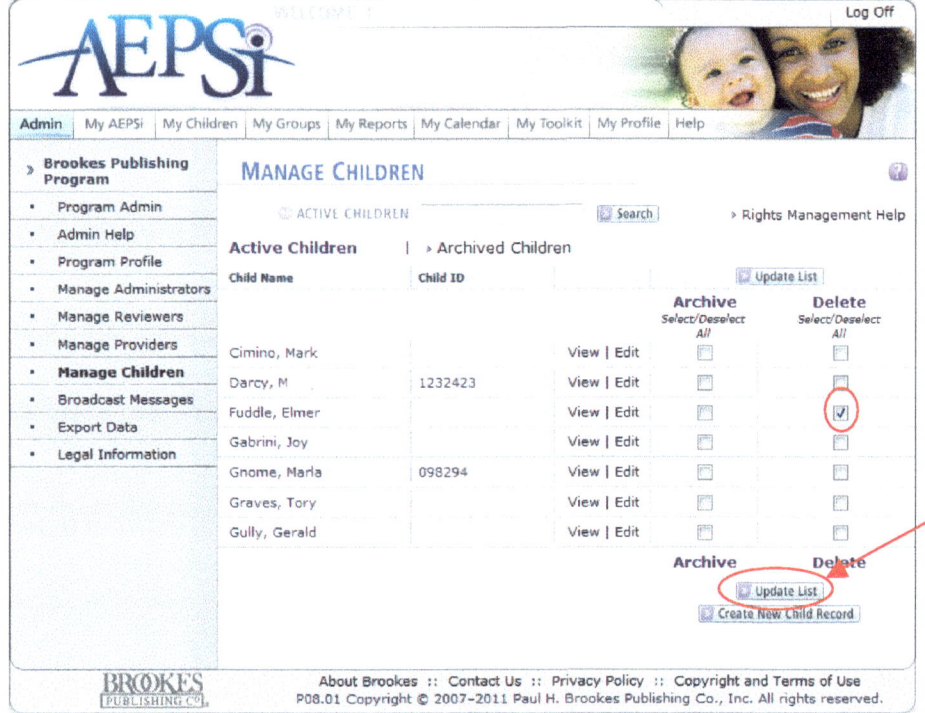

To delete child records, check the box(es) next to the child or children you would like to delete under the Delete column of either the Active Children or Archived Children sections of the **Manage Children** page.

You can also use the *Select/Deselect All* link to select all child records.

Click the *Update List* button.

The child records you have deleted will be completely removed from your account and will no longer be accessible.

My Reports

Section 4

AEPSi not only features powerful functions that make it easy to record, score, and track the AEPS Test but also enables you and your users to quickly generate status reports and build progress-over-time reports for an individual child and for groups of children.

AEPSi generates all of the paperwork for reports that otherwise would have to be created by hand: Score Summary, Graphed Scores, IFSP/IEP Summary, AEPS Child Progress Record, and Present Level of Functioning Report for use at IFSP/IEP meetings.

Coupled with the AEPS print manuals, AEPSi turns AEPS Test scores into OSEP Child Outcomes reports with a single click. You can be confident that your OSEP reports are reliable, valid, and exportable into any format your state requires. In another one-click report, you can compare a child's AEPS Test scores with rigorously researched cutoff scores to determine or corroborate a child's eligibility for services in most state systems.

In addition to creating individual Child, Class, and Program Reports, programs in the same district, region, or state can be linked so that Administrators can generate "roll-up" status and progress reports. We can even create custom reports for your state—just let us know your needs.

This section describes how to create individual reports for children, as well as Class and Program Reports, and provides more details on OSEP reporting and eligibility reports.

Child Reports

Child Reports are accessible to Providers and Administrators, as well as to Reviewers who have access to child identifying data. Providers can only create Child Reports for children they have been assigned to, whereas Administrators and Reviewers with access to child identifying data can view all Child Reports.

To run a Child Report for any child in your program, go to the **My Reports** section of AEPSi and click the *Child Reports* link.

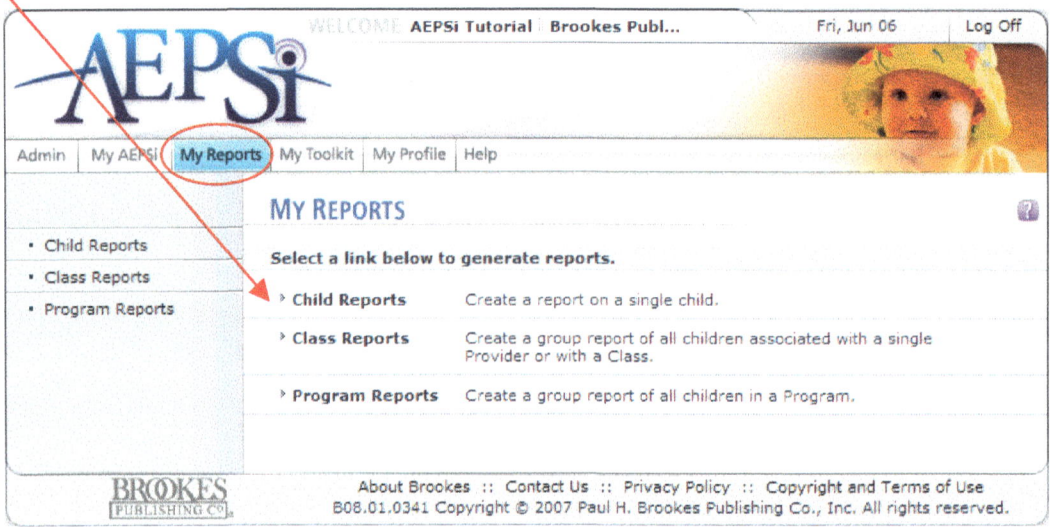

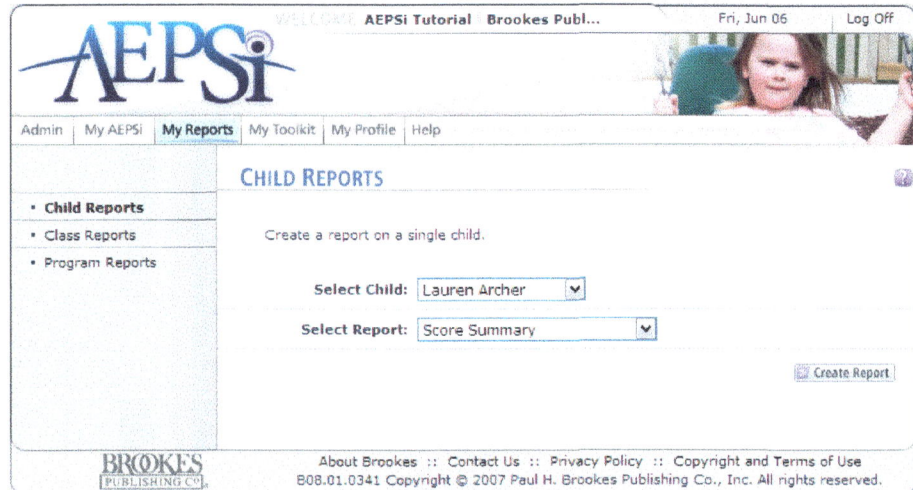

This will take you to the **Child Reports** page, where you can select which child and which report you would like to run from dropdown menus provided.

After selecting the child and report, click the *Create Report* button. You will be taken to a screen that allows you to select the test period for which to run the report.

After selecting the test period(s), click the *Create Report* button. The report will appear as a PDF, which you can then print or save directly to your computer.

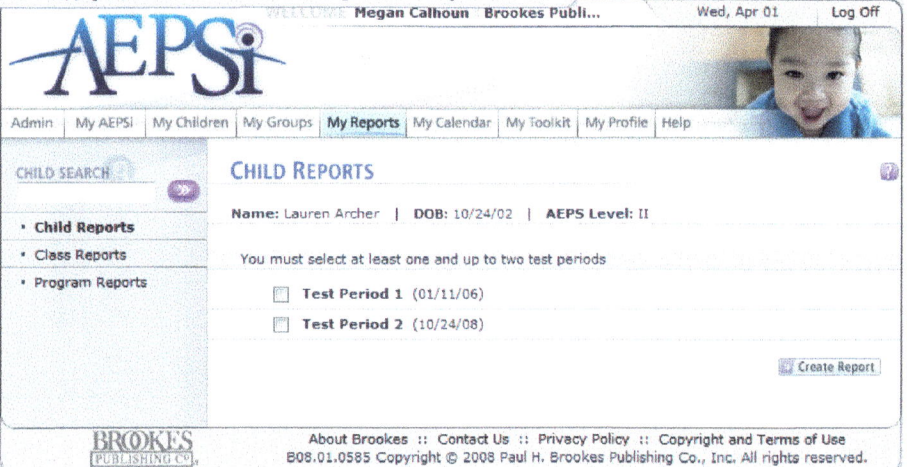

There are seven individual Child Reports to choose from in AEPSi.

Score Summary

The Score Summary displays the test date, raw score, possible raw score, and percent score for all six areas of the AEPS Test. Up to four test periods at a time display on one report.

AEPSi Administrator Guide | 35

Graphed Scores

Graphed Scores reports show bar graphs that represent a child's CODRF scores for different test periods. By comparing test periods as side-by-side bar graphs, you have a quick visual representation of a child's progress over time.

You can choose from the following reporting options:

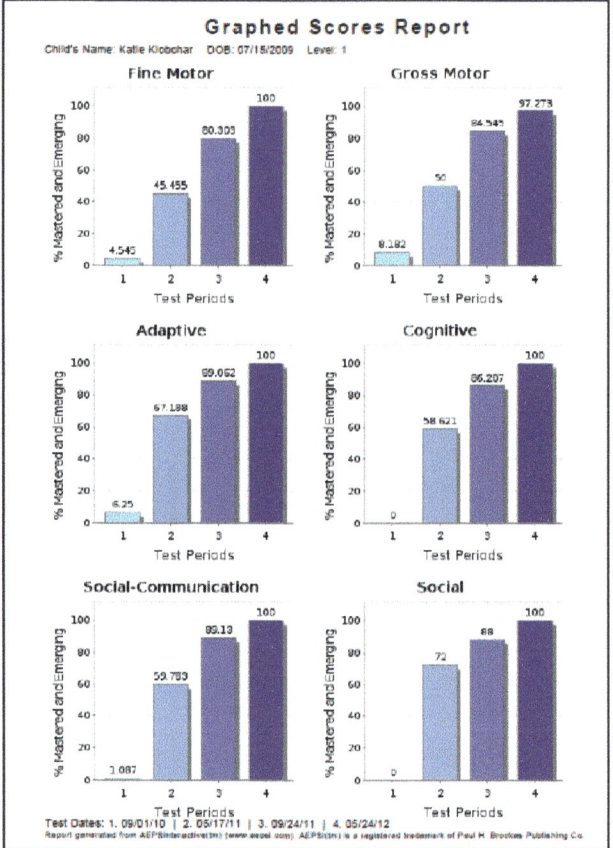

% of Mastered and Emerging (2 and 1): This report will add all items that were scored 1's and 2's and display the results as a percentage of the total score possible for each area.

% of Mastered (2): This report will add all items that were scored 2's and display the results as a percentage of the total score possible for each area.

% of Emerging (1): This report will add all items that were scored 1's and display the results as a percentage of the total score possible for each area.

% of Scoring Note A: This report shows you the percentage of items that had an accompanying scoring note of A for each area.

% of Scoring Note B: This report shows you the percentage of items that had an accompanying scoring note of B for each area.

% of Scoring Note M: This report shows you the percentage of items that had an accompanying scoring note of M for each area.

% of Scoring Note Q: This report shows you the percentage of items that had an accompanying scoring note of Q for each area.

% of Scoring Note R: This report shows you the percentage of items that had an accompanying scoring note of R for each area.

Child Progress Record

A Child Progress Record helps family members and Caregivers participate in the ongoing monitoring of their child's progress. The Child Progress Record offers a visual representation of a child's accomplishments, current targets, and future goals and objectives. As a child meets the standard criteria for a goal or objective, shading indicates the child's progress.

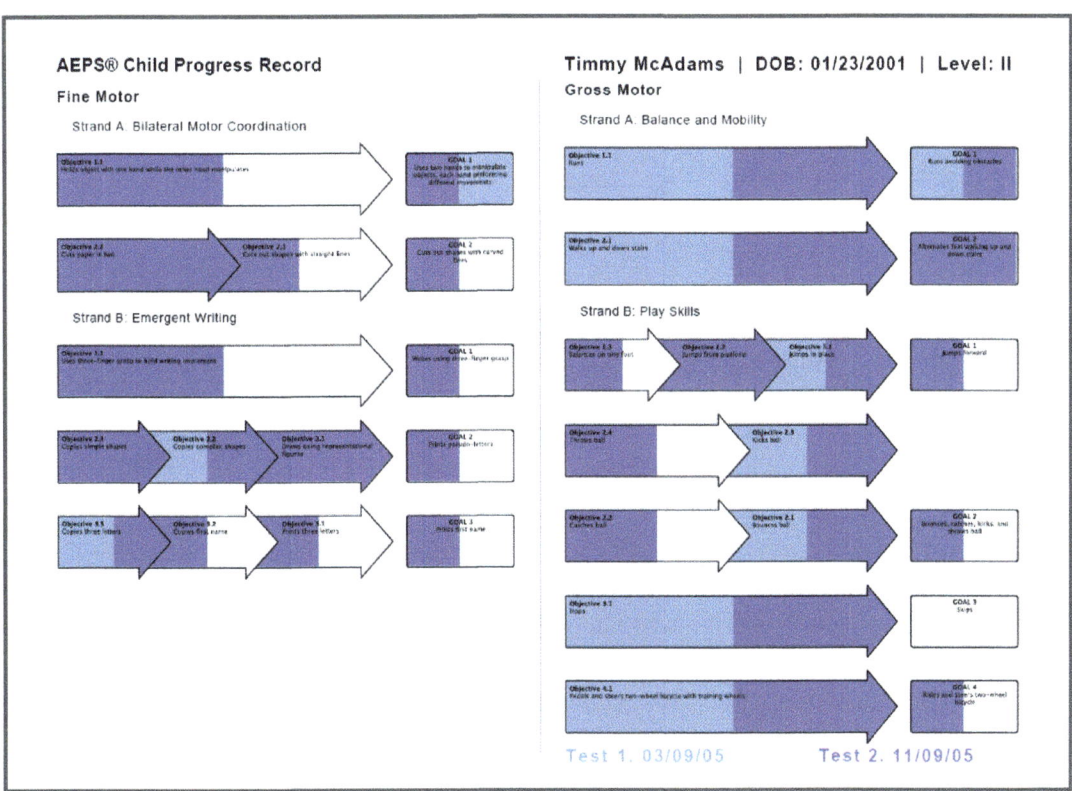

Provider Notes

The Provider Notes report displays any notes (A, B, D, M, Q, R) that were recorded in the CODRF for a child. This report displays the goal, the test item, the note, and any comments a Provider entered in the CODRF pertaining to the test item that had the note.

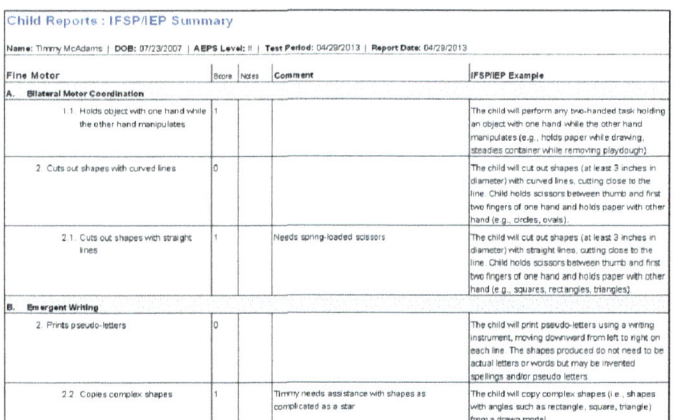

IFSP/IEP Summary

The IFSP/IEP Summary shows all items that had the IFSP/IEP box checked on an assessment. This report can be used to help in writing goals for a child's IFSP or IEP. The report also includes sample IFSP/IEP goals.

Eligibility Cutoff Scores Report

The Eligibility Cutoff Scores Report uses AEPS area scores to determine eligibility status. AEPSi automatically calculates the child's chronological age and compares area scores with empirically validated cutoff scores corresponding to the appropriate age interval. Extensive research shows that the cutoff scores are highly accurate in identifying children who are eligible for services, and the scores work well to corroborate findings of standardized, norm-referenced tests. If the child's area goal score is above the cutoff for a given area, the child's development is not delayed. If the child's area goal score is at or below the cutoff for a given area, his or her development is delayed.

For each area, the report displays test date, raw score, and cutoff score. At the end of the report, explanatory text is given concerning the AEPS cutoff scores and information about eligibility in the child's state.

Present Level of Functioning

The Present Level of Functioning report provides a summary of a child's AEPS Test results in terms of what skills are mastered (a score of 2), emerging (a score of 1), and not yet observed (a score of 0). Providers can use this report to write narrative reports for IFSP/IEP meetings.

Aggregate Reports

In addition to individual Child Reports, you can create aggregate reports of the children in your program.

These aggregate reports can be accessed by clicking either *Class Reports* or *Program Reports* from your **My Reports** page.

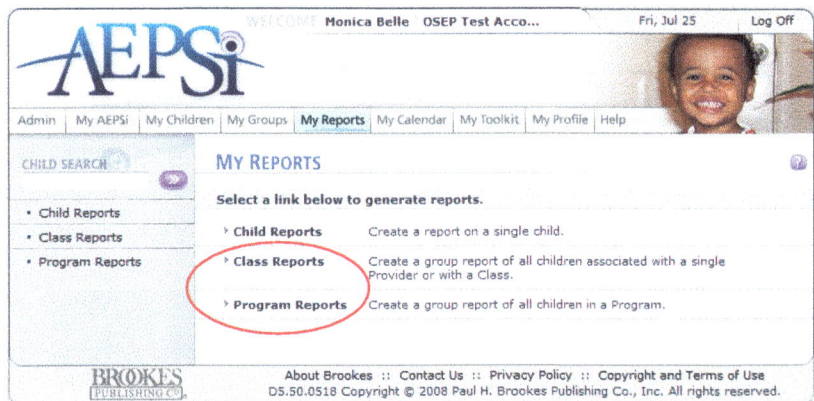

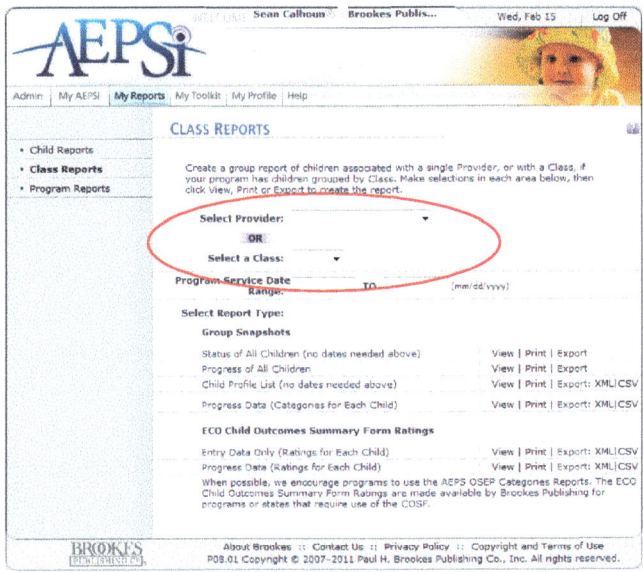

Class Reports Page

The **Class Reports** page allows you to run aggregate reports on children associated with a single Provider, or with a class if your program has children grouped by class.

To run a report based on Provider, simply select the name of the Provider from the dropdown menu of Providers. This menu will include all of the Providers who have been created in your program.

Likewise, when running a report based on a class, simply select the class from the dropdown menu of classrooms. This list will include all of the classrooms that have been created in your program's profile.

Program Reports Page

The **Program Reports** page allows you to run aggregate reports on all of the children in your program.

It looks very similar to the **Class Reports** page but does not have the options for selecting a Provider or a class at the top of the page.

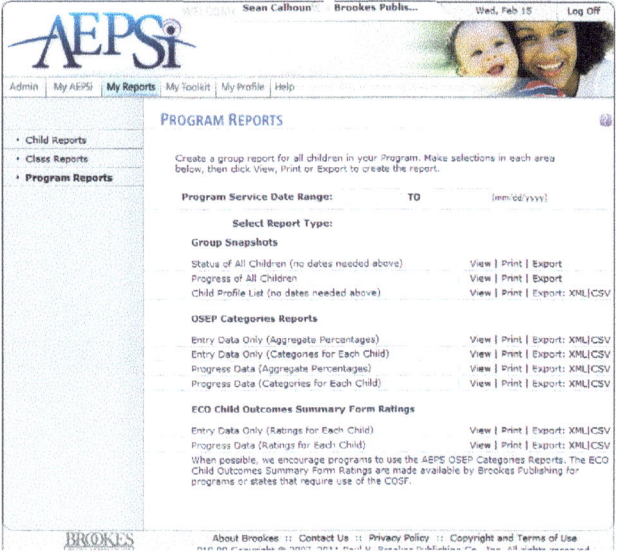

AEPSi Administrator Guide | 39

You can run three types of aggregate reports in AEPSi:
- Group Snapshot Reports
- OSEP Categories Reports
- ECO Child Outcome Summary Form Ratings

Group Snapshot Reports

Group Snapshots are reports that provide information on the assessment status, progress, and demographics of all active children under a Provider, within a class, or in the program. You can access three Group Snapshot reports: Status of All Children, Progress of All Children, and Child Profile List.

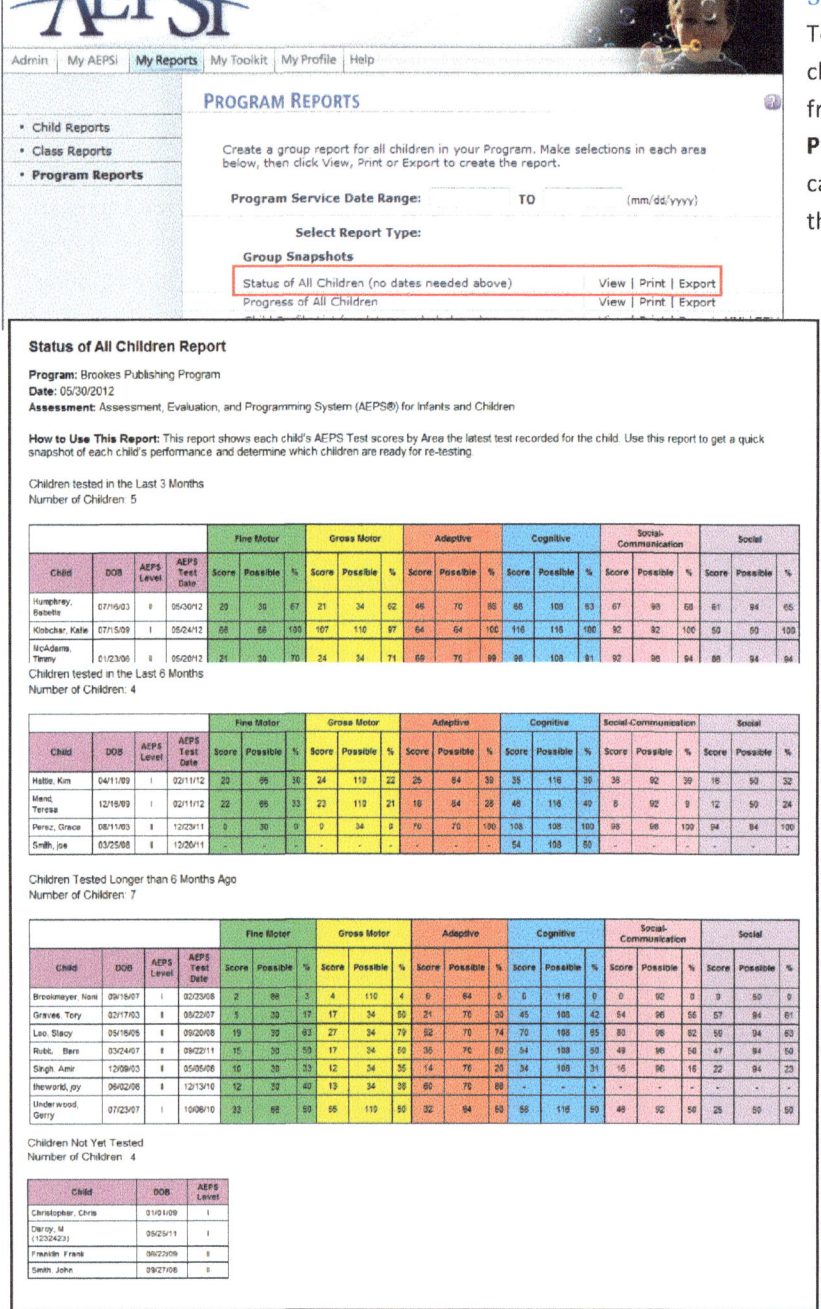

Status of All Children Report

To run a Status of All Children Report, click the *View* link next the report title from either the **Class Reports** or the **Program Reports** pages. The report can also be printed or exported from these pages.

The Status of All Children Report shows each child's AEPS assessment scores, possible score, and a percentage score for each of the six Areas on that child's most recent assessment. Children are grouped into 4 categories:

- Those tested in the last 3 months
- Those tested in the last 6 months
- Those tested longer than 6 months ago
- Those not yet tested

This report gives you a quick look at how all of the children are performing and helps you determine which children are ready for retesting.

Progress of All Children Report

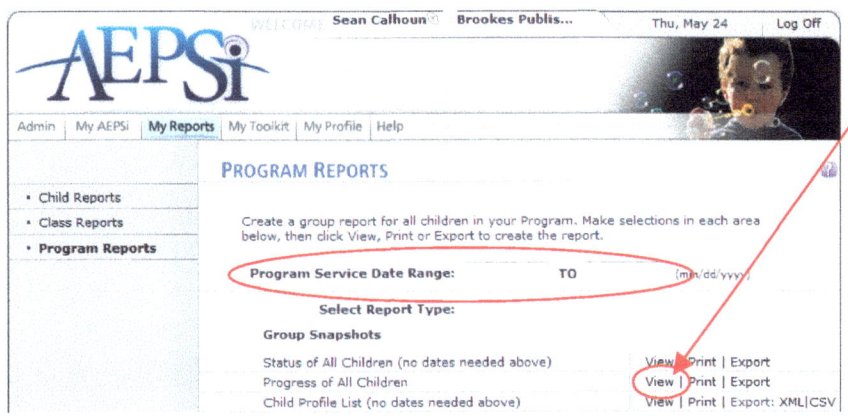

To run a Progress of All Children Report, enter the service date range for which you would like to run the report, then click the *View* link next to the report title from either the **Class Reports** or the **Program Reports** pages. This report can also be printed or exported from these pages.

The Progress of All Children Report shows each child's AEPS assessment scores by Area for the first and last test recorded for the child during the date range selected, and calculates the increase or decrease between the two assessments.

The report also provides a list of each skill that has been mastered, is emerging, or has not been observed.

Children who do not have two test periods within the date range selected will be listed at the bottom of the report.

This report gives you a quick look at each child's progress over time and which skills the child still needs to develop.

AEPSi Administrator Guide | 41

Child Profile List Report

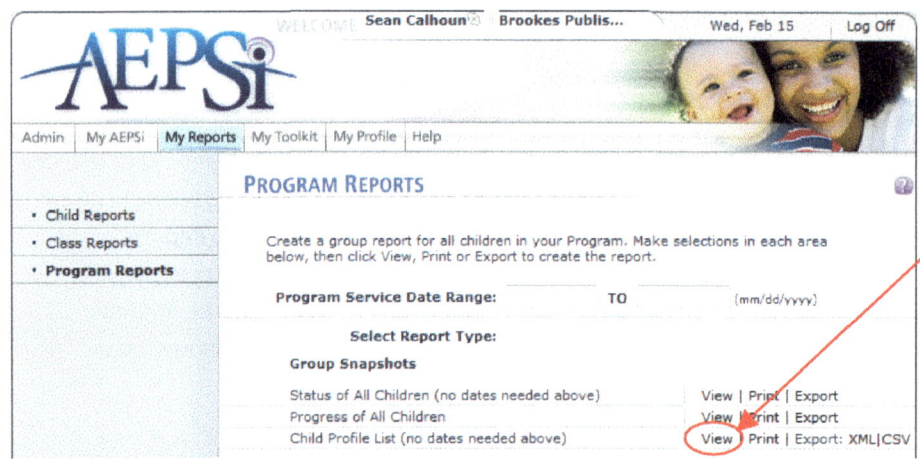

To run a Child Profile List Report, click the *View* link next the report title from the **Class Reports** or **Program Reports** page.

The Child Profile List Report contains the demographic information for all children, both active and archived. The report includes the following:

- Child Name and Child ID
- Child DOB
- Child Status (Active or Archived)
- Gender
- Classroom
- Developmental Status
- Lead Provider
- AEPS level
- Include in OSEP Reporting (Yes or No)
- Funding Source
- Program Entry Date
- Program Exit Date
- Recent Assessment Status

The exported versions of the report (XML or CSV) contain additional useful information, including archived date, number of assessments, and any custom fields that have been created.

OSEP Categories Reports

About OSEP Reporting

OSEP reporting is easy with AEPSi, which automatically transforms AEPS Test results using the crosswalk of AEPS items with the three OSEP Child Outcomes and empirically derived same-age-peer benchmarks. Because AEPS's crosswalk correlated to OSEP Child Outcomes has been empirically validated, you can rest assured that child outcomes data reported with AEPSi are accurate and genuine measures of OSEP Child Outcomes. With reliable child outcomes data, Providers can better tailor interventions to children's needs, and you can be confident that entry and exit data will show progress.

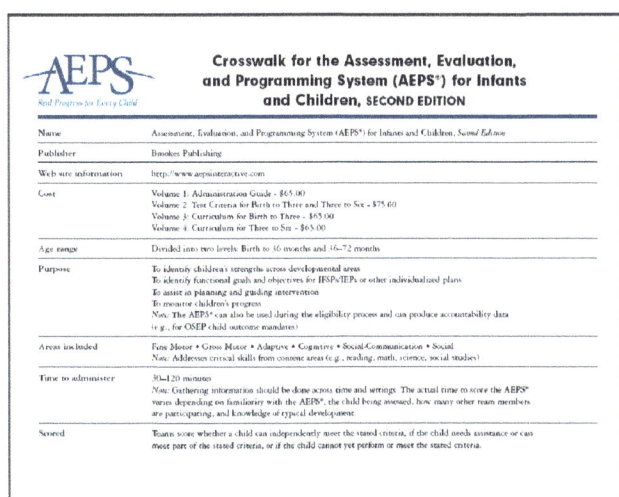

To generate the OSEP report, AEPSi:

1. Calculates each child's OSEP Outcomes raw scores by gathering and summing children's scores on the specific AEPS Test items that correlate to the three child outcomes required by OSEP
2. Shows whether a child is performing at the level of same-age peers. Outcome raw scores are compared to empirically validated same-age-peer benchmarks at the appropriate age intervals. Raw scores at or above the benchmarks indicate that a child's performance is similar to same-age peers. Raw scores below the benchmarks indicate that a child's performance is below that of same-age peers.
3. Sorts children into two categories at near entry:
    - Performing as same-age peers
    - Not performing as same-age peers
4. Sorts children into five categories at near exit:
    - Maintained functioning at a level comparable to same-age peers
    - Improved functioning to reach a level comparable to same-age peers
    - Improved functioning to a level nearer to same-age peers but did not reach comparable level
    - Improved functioning but not sufficient to move nearer to functioning comparable to same-age peers
    - Did not improve functioning

There are four OSEP Categories reports that are available in a viewable, printable, and exportable format. The reports are automatically separated by Part B and Part C.

- Entry Data Only (Aggregate Percentages)
- Entry Data Only (Categories for Each Child)
- Progress Data (Aggregate Percentages)
- Progress Data (Categories for Each Child)

Note: Even though you are no longer required to submit entry data to OSEP, AEPSi still has two entry data reports, which are helpful in determining where children enter the program and monitoring whether children received their entry assessments—which are needed in order to report on progress.

Children on the Alternative Path

Children who are 37 months or older and are still using the Level I test due to severe developmental disabilities are automatically placed on the alternative path for OSEP reporting. At near entry, these children will have an OSEP Outcome of not performing as same-age peers. Based on an alternative method, AEPSi will generate OSEP Outcomes and recommended ECO ratings. On the Raw Score reports, the raw score and same-age benchmark will be displayed as "n/a."

Roberts, Damien	09375	07/09/03	09/01/06	10/13/06	n/a	n/a	B	n/a	n/a	B	n/a	n/a	B

There is nothing a user needs to do in order to place a child on the alternative path. If the child is 37 months or older and a Level I test was used to assess the child, that child will automatically be placed on the alternative path.

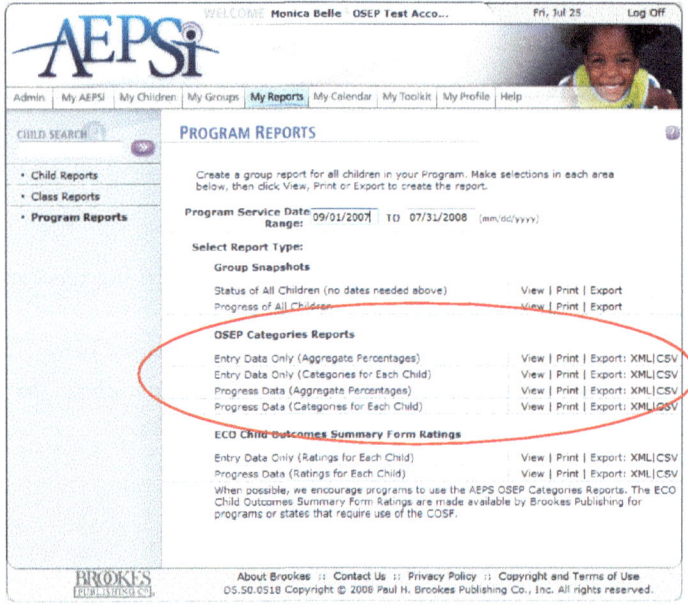

All of the OSEP Categories reports can be run from either the **Class Reports** page or the **Program Reports** page by entering a service date range and then clicking on the *View* link next to the report you would like to run.

All OSEP Categories reports can also be printed from these pages or exported into XML or CSV files.

Entry Data Only (Aggregate Percentages) Report

The Entry Data Only (Aggregate Percentages) report calculates each child's OSEP Outcomes raw scores, compares them to same-age-peer benchmarks, and aggregates the results for each of the three OSEP Child Outcomes.

The report displays the percentage of children who are performing at a level comparable to same-age peers and the percentage of children who are not performing at a level comparable to same-age peers.

The results are separated by Part B and Part C, according to the funding source that was selected in the child's profile.

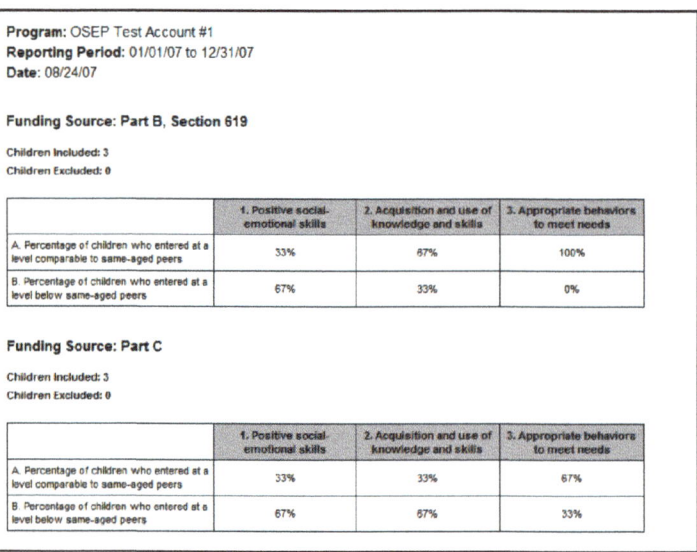

The report also displays the number of children who were included in the report and the number of children who were excluded. More details on why children were excluded from the report are shown in the Entry Data Only (Categories for Each Child) report.

Entry Data Only (Categories for Each Child) Report

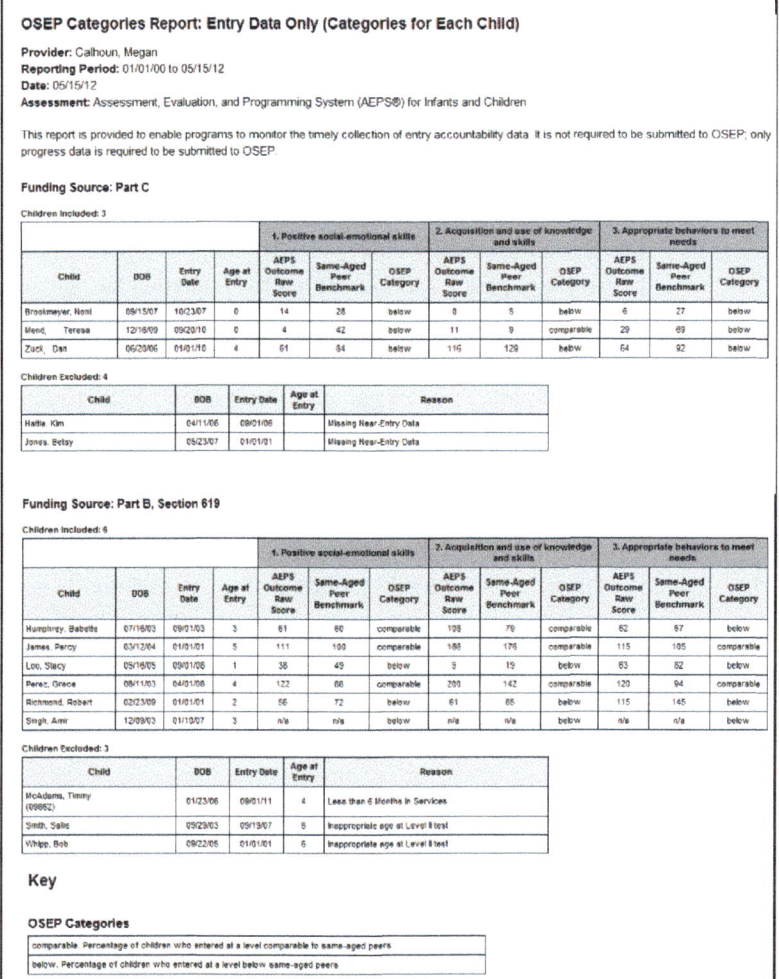

The Entry Data Only (Categories for Each Child) report calculates and displays each child's OSEP Outcomes raw scores for the three OSEP Child Outcomes, the corresponding same-age-peer benchmarks, and whether the child is below or comparable to same-age peers.

In addition, the report displays the child's name, date of birth, program entry date, and age at entry (measured in years).

The report is separated by Part B and Part C.

A list of children who were excluded from the report and the reason why is also included.

In addition, the export versions of the report (XML and CSV) include any custom fields that have been created.

Progress Data (Aggregate Percentages) Report

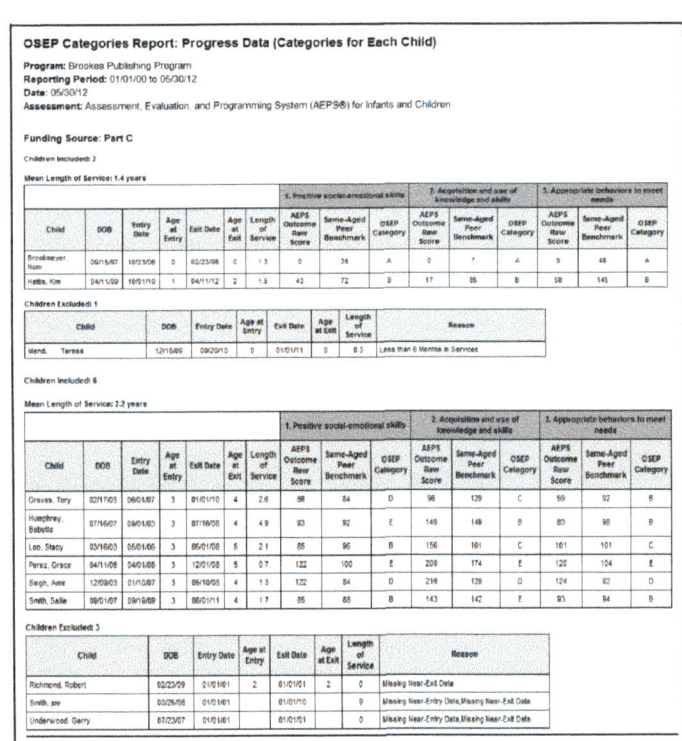

The Progress Data (Aggregate Percentages) report calculates each child's OSEP Outcomes raw scores, compares them to their near-entry raw scores and/or same-age-peer benchmarks, and aggregates the results for each of the three OSEP Child Outcomes.

The report displays the percentage of children at near exit who maintained functioning at a level comparable to same-age peers, improved functioning to reach a level comparable to same-age peers, improved functioning to a level nearer to same-age peers but did not reach a comparable level, improved functioning but not sufficient to move nearer to functioning comparable to same-age peers, and did not improve functioning.

The results are separated by Part B and Part C, according to the funding source that was selected in the child profile.

The report also displays the number of children who were included in the report and the number of children who were excluded. More information on excluded children is included in the Progress Data (Categories for Each Child) report.

Progress Data (Categories for Each Child) Report

The Progress Data (Categories for Each Child) report calculates and displays each child's OSEP Outcomes raw scores for the three OSEP Child Outcomes, the corresponding same-age-peer benchmarks, and the OSEP Category.

In addition, the report displays the child's name, date of birth, program entry date, age at entry, program exit date, age at exit, and length of service.

The report is separated by Part B and Part C.

A list of children who were excluded from the report and the reason why is also included. In addition, the export versions of the report include any custom fields.

OSEP Report Exclusion Categories

A child may be excluded from an OSEP report due to several reasons. Below is a list of the exclusion categories and instructions on what your Providers need to do to correct the errors.

Missing Near-Entry Data:

Children Excluded:

Child	ID	DOB	Entry Date	Exit Date	Reason
Abaiye, Oni		07/11/05	10/23/07	10/23/08	Missing Near-Entry Data

Either the near-entry assessment has not been selected for a child or it has not been finalized.

What to do: Make sure a near-entry assessment has been selected for the child. Also, the Provider should verify that the assessment has been finalized and that all test items are complete. If another assessment tool was used to assess a child at near entry, the online COSF (Child Outcomes Summary Form) can be used in place of an AEPS assessment.

Missing Near-Exit Data:

Children Excluded:

Child	ID	DOB	Entry Date	Exit Date	Reason
Butterfield, Marcy		12/21/03	09/01/04	05/21/08	Missing Near-Exit Data

Either the near-exit assessment has not been selected for a child or it has not been finalized.

What to do: Make sure a near-exit assessment has been selected for the child. Also, the Provider should verify that the assessment has been finalized and that all test items are complete.

Less than 6 Months in Services:

Children Excluded:

Child	ID	DOB	Entry Date	Exit Date	Reason
Archer, Lauren	19832	12/15/02	12/16/05	03/01/06	Less than 6 Months in Services

There are less than 6 months between the child's program entry and program exit date. OSEP has mandated that only children who have received services for at least 6 months should be reported.

What to do: Go to the child's profile page and verify that the correct program entry and program exit dates have been entered. If the correct dates are entered and there are still less than 6 months of services received, this child should be excluded from OSEP reporting.

Invalid Funding Source:

Children Excluded:

Child	ID	DOB	Entry Date	Exit Date	Reason
Archer, Lauren	19832	12/15/02	12/16/05	07/01/07	Invalid Funding Source

A funding source other than Part B or Part C has been selected for the child.

What to do: Verify that either Part B or Part C has been selected for funding source on the child's profile page.

Inappropriate Age at Level II Test:

Children Excluded:

Child	ID	DOB	Entry Date	Exit Date	Reason
Archer, Lauren	19832	12/15/00	12/16/05	07/01/07	Inappropriate age at Level II test

If a child is 36 months or younger and is using a Level II test, the inappropriate test was used to assess the child. A Level II test should be used only once a child is older than 36 months and is in the Part B program.

What to do: Assess the child with the age-appropriate test.

ECO Child Outcomes Summary Form Ratings

There are two ECO Child Outcomes Summary Form Ratings, one with near-entry data only and one with progress data.

These reports can be run from either the **Class Reports** or the **Program Reports** pages by entering the service date range and then clicking on the *View* link next to the report you would like to run.

The ECO Child Outcomes Summary Form Ratings can also be printed from these pages or exported into either XML or CSV files.

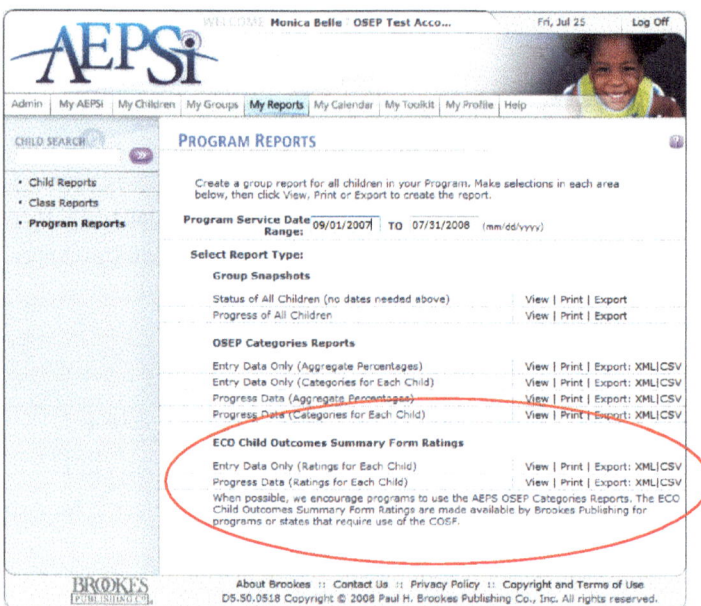

Entry Data Only (Ratings for Each Child) Report

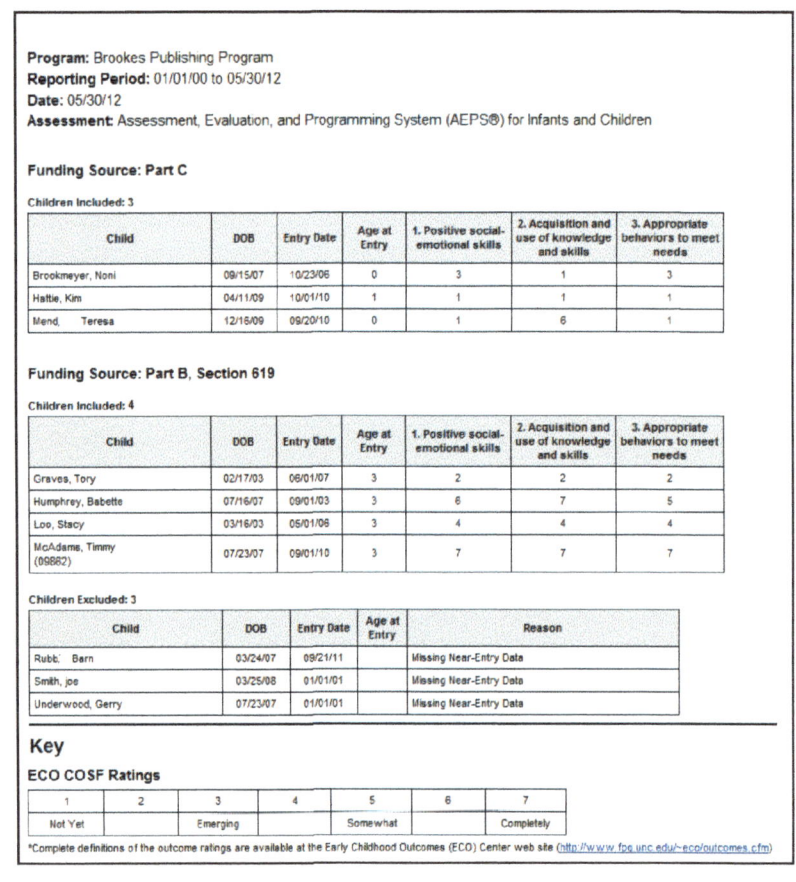

For those programs that require use of the COSF, AEPSi provides a recommended ECO Rating for each child using the 1 to 7 scale. The report displays the child's name, date of birth, program entry date, age at entry, and the recommended ECO rating for each of the three outcomes.

The report also includes a list of children who were excluded and the reasons why.

48 | AEPSi Administrator Guide

Progress Data (Ratings for Each Child) Report

ECO Child Outcomes Summary Form Ratings: Progress Data (Ratings for Each Child)

Program: Brookes Publishing Program
Reporting Period: 01/01/00 to 06/04/12
Date: 06/04/12
Assessment: Assessment, Evaluation, and Programming System (AEPS®) for Infants and Children

Funding Source: Part C

Children Included: 2

Mean Length of Service: 1.4 years

Child	DOB	Entry Date	Age at Entry	Exit Date	Age at Exit	Length of Service	1. Positive social-emotional skills			2. Acquisition and use of knowledge and skills			3. Appropriate behaviors to meet needs		
							Entry	Exit	Progress	Entry	Exit	Progress	Entry	Exit	Progress
Brookmeyer, Noni	08/15/07	10/23/08	0	02/23/08	0	1.3	3	1	N	1	1	N	3	1	N
Hattie, Kim	04/11/09	10/01/10	1	04/11/12	2	1.5	1	1	Y	1	1	Y	1	1	Y

Children Excluded: 1

Child	DOB	Entry Date	Age at Entry	Exit Date	Age at Exit	Length of Service	Reason
Mend, Teresa	12/16/09	09/20/10	0	01/01/11	0	0.3	Less than 6 Months in Services

Funding Source: Part B, Section 619

Children Included: 7

Mean Length of Service: 2.1 years

Child	DOB	Entry Date	Age at Entry	Exit Date	Age at Exit	Length of Service	1. Positive social-emotional skills			2. Acquisition and use of knowledge and skills			3. Appropriate behaviors to meet needs		
							Entry	Exit	Progress	Entry	Exit	Progress	Entry	Exit	Progress
Graves, Tory	02/17/03	06/01/07	3	01/01/10	4	2.6	2	6	Y	2	4	Y	2	2	Y
Humphrey, Babette	07/16/07	09/01/03	3	07/16/05	4	4.9	6	6	Y	7	5	Y	5	4	Y
Lee, Stacy	03/16/03	05/01/06	3	06/01/08	5	2.1	4	4	Y	4	5	Y	4	5	Y
Perez, Grace	04/11/06	04/01/08	3	12/01/08	5	0.7	7	7	Y	7	7	Y	7	7	Y
Singh, Amir	12/09/03	01/10/07	3	05/10/08	4	1.3	1	7	Y	1	7	Y	1	7	Y
Smith, Sallie	09/01/07	09/19/09	3	06/01/11	4	1.7	7	5	Y	7	6	Y	5	5	Y
Zuck, Dan	06/20/06	10/01/10	4	05/31/12	5	1.7	3	7	Y	5	7	Y	2	6	Y

Children Excluded: 3

Child	DOB	Entry Date	Age at Entry	Exit Date	Age at Exit	Length of Service	Reason
Richmond, Robert	02/23/08	01/01/01	2	01/01/01	2	0	Missing Near-Exit Data
Smith, Joe	03/25/08	01/01/01		01/01/10		9	Missing Near-Entry Data, Missing Near-Exit Data
Underwood, Gerry	07/23/07	01/01/01		01/01/01		0	Missing Near-Entry Data, Missing Near-Exit Data

Key

ECO COSF Ratings

1	2	3	4	5	6	7
Not Yet		Emerging		Somewhat		Completely

*Complete definitions of the outcome ratings are available at the Early Childhood Outcomes (ECO) Center web site (http://www.fpg.unc.edu/~ecoioutcomes.cfm)

The Progress Data (Ratings for Each Child) report displays the recommended ECO ratings for near entry and near exit and indicates whether progress occurred (Y for yes, N for no).

Also included in the report are the child's name, date of birth, program entry date, age at entry, program exit date, age at exit, and the length of service (measured in years).

A list of children who were excluded from the report and the reasons why is displayed as well.

Broadcast Messages

Section 5

As Administrator, you have the ability to create messages that will be displayed on the My AEPSi home page for all users in your program.

Creating a Message

To create a message:

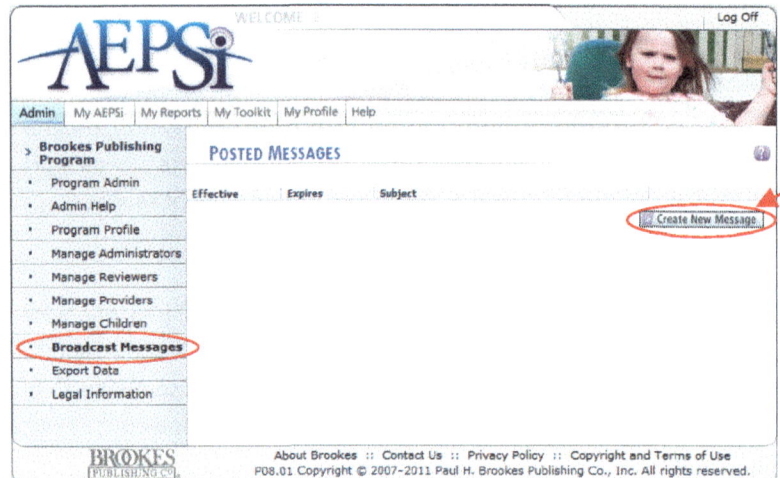

Click on the **Admin** tab, and select the *Broadcast Messages* link from the left menu navigation.

Click the *Create New Message* button.

This will take you to the **Create/Edit Message** page.

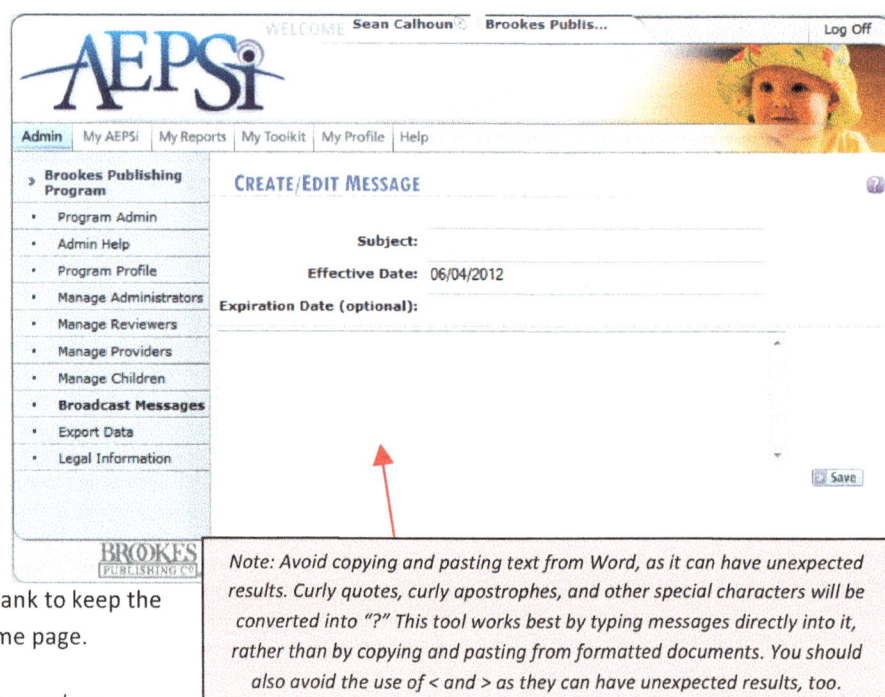

From the **Create/Edit Message** page, enter a subject for your message. Enter the effective date for your message. The default date will be today's date. This is the date your message will begin to appear on the **My AEPSi** home page.

You have the option to enter an expiration date for a message. Once a message has expired it will no longer appear on the **My AEPSi** home page. Leave this field blank to keep the message displayed on the home page.

Note: Avoid copying and pasting text from Word, as it can have unexpected results. Curly quotes, curly apostrophes, and other special characters will be converted into "?" This tool works best by typing messages directly into it, rather than by copying and pasting from formatted documents. You should also avoid the use of < and > as they can have unexpected results, too.

Type your message in the text area box.

Click the *Save* button.

Viewing/Editing/Deleting a Message

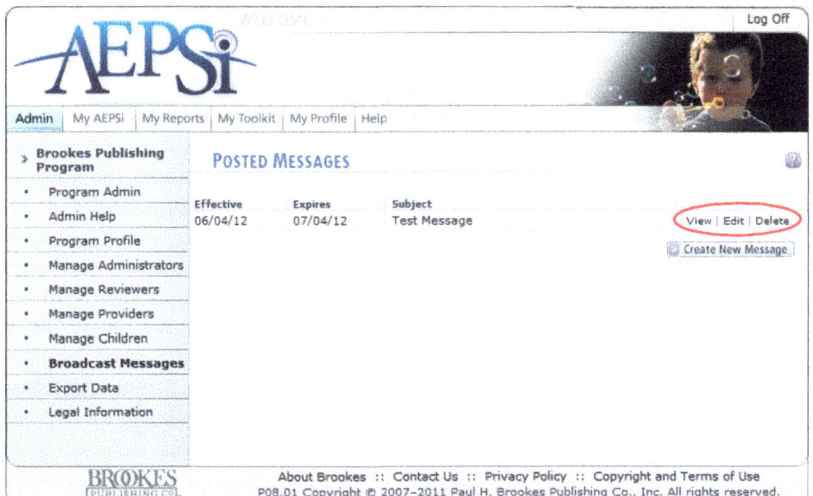

To view, edit, or delete a message, click the *View*, *Edit*, or *Delete* links next to the message for which you would like to perform these actions from the **Broadcast Messages** page.

Deleting a message will permanently remove the message from your list of Posted Messages and from the **My AEPSi** home page of all users.

Adding a Hyperlink to a Message

You also have the ability to include hyperlinks in the text of your message. When users select the hyperlink, the website will appear in an Internet browser window.

To add a hyperlink to a message, insert a hash mark (#) before and after the hyperlink.

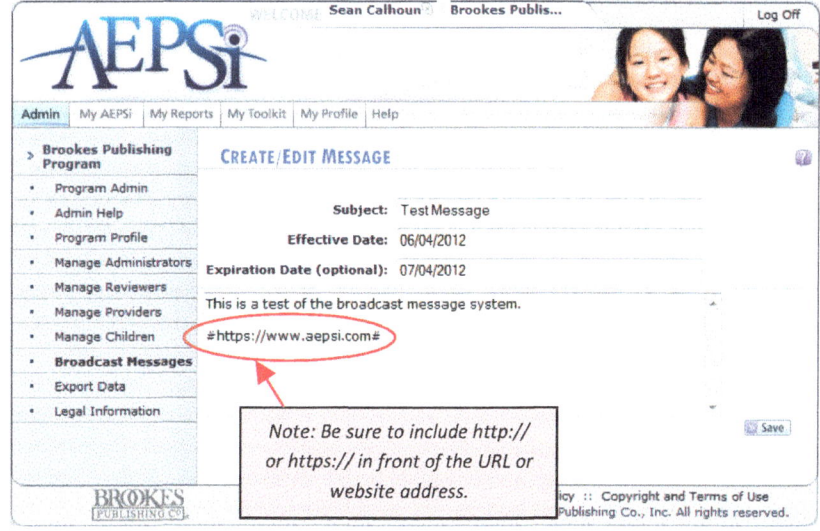

Exporting Data

Section 6

Export Child Data

Your program owns any data that are entered and generated in AEPSi. You may export all or part of the data at any time. We are committed to using standards-based formats for exporting data so that programs can easily export data for use in other databases. A child's assessments and reports can be exported individually by Providers via links on the **Child Summary** page. If your program needs custom services, contact your implementation manager at implementation@brookespublishing.com.

To export data for one or more children, click on the *Export Data* link on the left navigation menu, select the name(s) of the children you would like to export, and click the *Export Data* button.

The following child data will be exported: child profile data, Caregiver profile(s), child journal, and child assessment data.

The format of the export is XML (Extensible Markup Language). XML is a flexible language that can be used to import data into other databases and can be converted to other text formats.

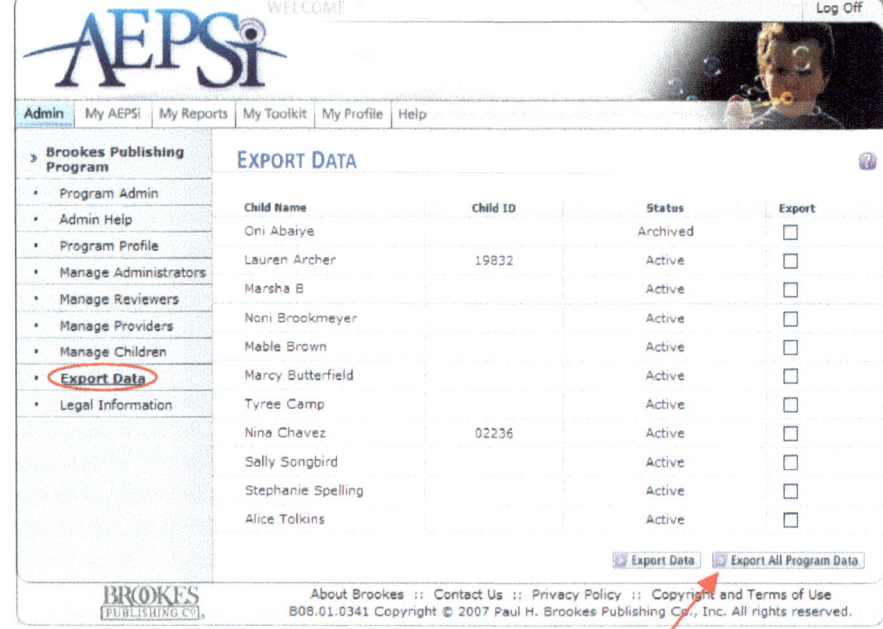

Export Program Data

You also have the option to export your entire program's data. Clicking *Export All Program Data* will export data for all children, including child profile data, Caregiver profile(s), child journals, and child assessment data. The format for the program data export is XML.

Support and Training

Section 7

Password Management

As Administrator, you can give members of your organization access to AEPSi at no extra charge. Subscription charges are based on the number of child records, not the number of users.

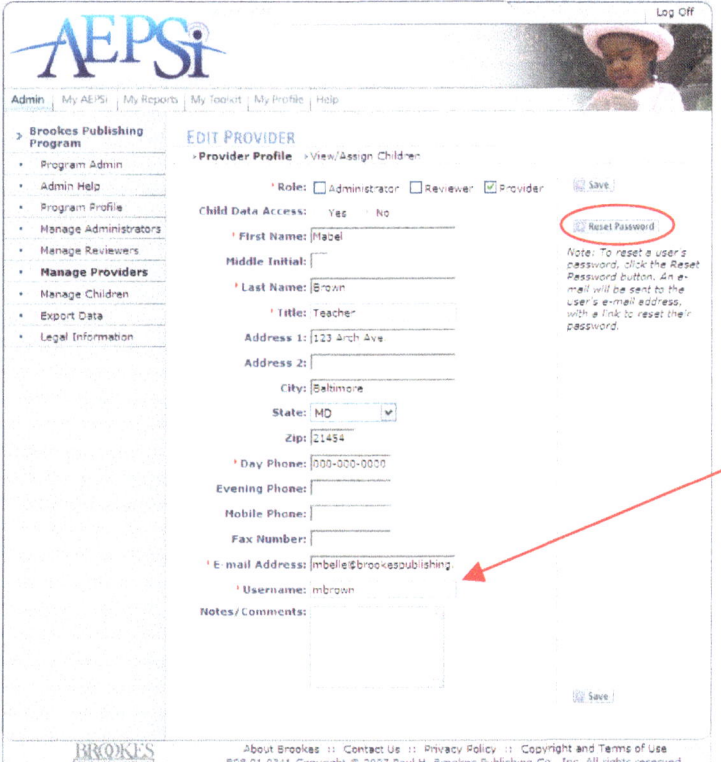

Forgotten Passwords

All users can reset a forgotten password by using the *Forgot Password?* link on the login page, provided they know their usernames. As Administrator, you can reset a user's password by clicking the reset password button in his or her user profile. An e-mail will be sent to the user with a secure link. When the user selects the link, he or she will be directed to a page to enter a new password.

Forgotten Username

Users who have forgotten their usernames can select the *Forgot Username?* link on the login page. As Administrator, you can access the user's profile and provide his or her username.

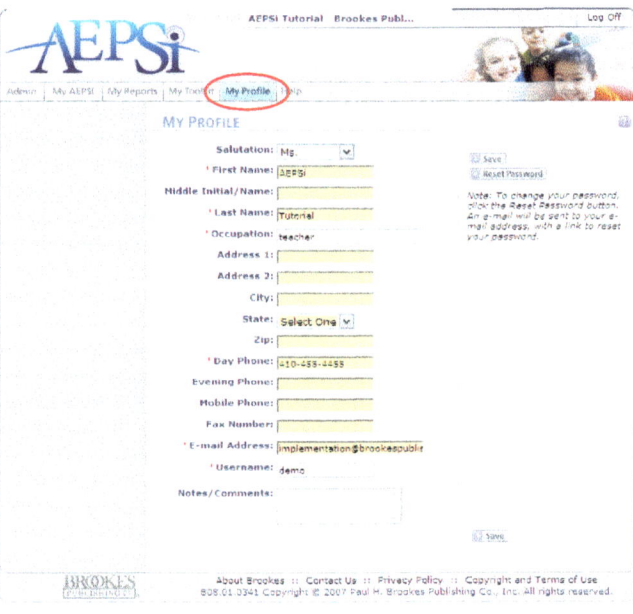

Change Password

You can change your password in the **My Profile** section of AEPSi.
1. Select My Profile from the top menu.
2. Click the *Reset Password* button.
3. An e-mail will be sent to you with a secure link. When you select the link, you will be directed to a page where you will be asked to enter a new password.

Password Protection

For security reasons, you should never share your username and/or password with anyone. A professional at your organization who needs to use AEPSi or access AEPSi data should be given his or her own username and password.

AEPSi Administrator Guide | 53

Technical Support

Technical Support is available 24/7 and is included with your subscription. You can reach technical support via phone, 1-866-386-2666 ext. 1, or e-mail, techsupport@brookespublishing.com.

My Toolkit

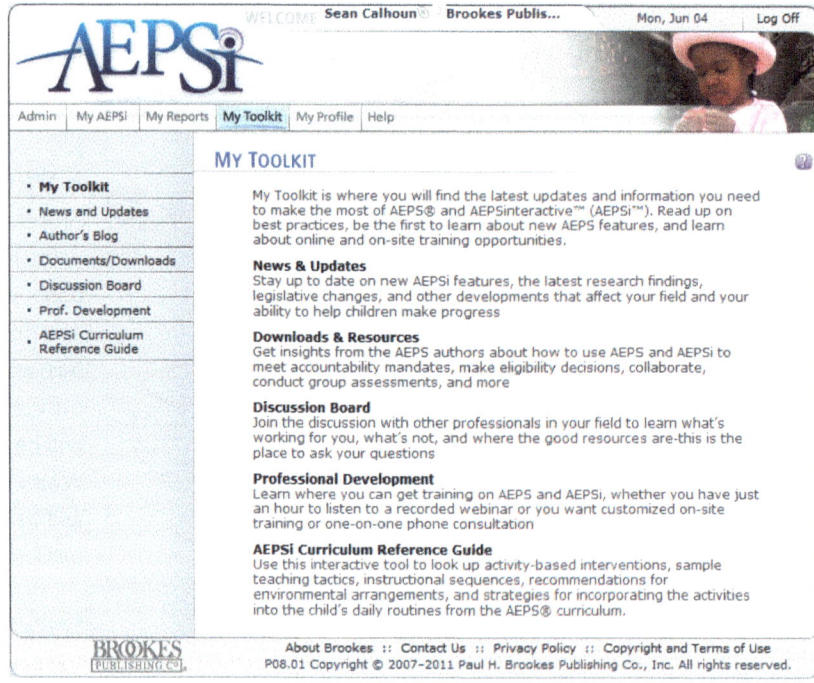

My Toolkit is where you can find updates and new information relating to AEPS and AEPSi. Here you will be able to find everything from the latest news and updates from Brookes Publishing Co. and the authors of AEPS to resources for professional development and training.

In the **News & Updates** section, you can find announcements, updates, and bug fixes related to the AEPSi application.

The **Downloads & Resources** section contains a collection of useful documents as well as other downloadable resources.

Also available is a **Discussion Board,** where users across states and sites can communicate, share ideas, and ask questions relating to both AEPS and AEPSi.

In the **Professional Development** section, you can find detailed information about content consulting, live training, and web-based training options, including webcasts and webinars.

In the **AEPSi Curriculum Reference Guide** section, you can access interactive tools that allow you to locate activity-based interventions, sample teaching tactics, instructional sequences, recommendations for environmental arrangements, and strategies for incorporating the activities into the children's daily routines from the AEPS curriculum.

Online Help and Support

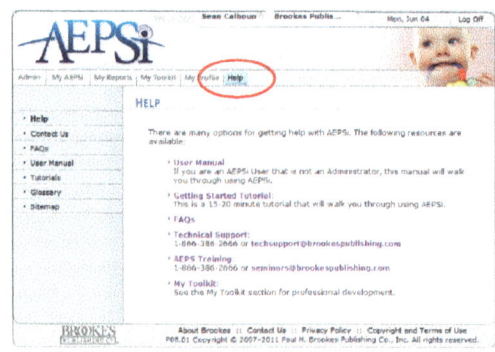

There are several online help and support resources to provide assistance to you and the registered users of your AEPSi account. Self-guided online tutorials are always accessible for Administrators and Providers. There is an extensive and regularly updated FAQ section available online.

Training

Customized On-Site Training

We want to ensure that you and your program staff members are knowledgeable and comfortable using AEPS and AEPSi. We provide a range of training options, including:

- Customized on-site seminars
- Web-based seminars
- Self-guided tutorials, and
- One-on-one telephone consultation

All training is conducted by experienced AEPS experts.

Training to Match Your Needs
We will work with you to arrive at the right mix of training for your program. Your staff's level of experience, the age range of children served, program size, budget, and schedule are all taken into consideration.

How Much Training Do You Need?
For first-time AEPS users, we recommend 2 days of customized on-site training on how to use the system for assessment and intervention. Additional half-day sessions are recommended for programs interested in using AEPS for OSEP reporting or eligibility determination. All on-site seminars are customizable; we can dedicate all or a portion of the sessions to "training the trainers," and we can adapt the topics to the needs of the program.

Pricing for On-Site Seminars
Fees vary depending on speaker experience, audience size, travel involved, and planning time; speaker's travel expenses and any required materials are additional.

AEPSi Training Options
Once you are familiar with AEPS, learning to use AEPSi is simple and straightforward. AEPSi users receive extensive support with their subscriptions:

- An introductory web-based seminar (for Administrators)
- Free self-guided tutorials
- Free access to 24/7 Technical Support
- Online user's manuals and FAQs

You can also work with our implementation team to customize AEPSi webinars for your program.